Rheumatoi

YOUR QUESTIONS A

G000066593

Commissioning Editor: Ellen Green
Project Development Manager: Isobel Black
Project Manager: Frances Affleck
Design Direction: George Ajayi

Rheumatoid arthritis

YOUR QUESTIONS ANSWERED

Robert J Moots
BSc(Hons) (LOND) MBBS(Hons) (LOND) PhD FRCP (LOND)
Professor of Rheumatology, University of Liverpool, University Hospital Aintree,
Liverpool, UK

Nigel Jones
MB ChB DipSEM
General Practitioner, Aintree Park Group Practice; Hospital Practitioner in
Musculoskeletal Medicine, University Hospital Aintree, Liverpool, UK

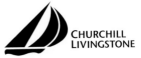

CHURCHILL
LIVINGSTONE

EDINBURGH LONDON NEW YORK OXFORD PHILADELPHIA ST LOUIS SYDNEY TORONTO 2004

CHURCHILL LIVINGSTONE
An imprint of Elsevier Limited

First published 2004

ISBN 0 443 07442 9

British Library Cataloguing in Publication Data
A catalogue record for this book is available from the British Library

Library of Congress Cataloging in Publication Data
A catalog record for this book is available from the Library of Congress

Notice
Medical knowledge is constantly changing. Standard safety precautions must be followed, but as new research and clinical experience broaden our knowledge, changes in treatment and drug therapy may become necessary or appropriate. Readers are advised to check the most current product information provided by the manufacturer of each drug to be administered to verify the recommended dose, the method and duration of administration, and contraindications. It is the responsibility of the practitioner, relying on experience and knowledge of the patient, to determine dosages and the best treatment for each individual patient. Neither the Publisher nor the authors assume any liability for any injury and/or damage to persons or property arising from this publication.
The Publisher

your source for books,
journals and multimedia
in the health sciences
www.elsevierhealth.com

The
publisher's
policy is to use
**paper manufactured
from sustainable forests**

Printed in China

Contents

Preface

Rheumatoid arthritis (RA) is one of the most common autoimmune diseases, affecting more than 1% of the population of the United Kingdom. Rheumatoid arthritis can affect individuals of almost any age and, even now, is a cause of significant disability. Furthermore, rheumatoid arthritis has been shown to be associated with a significantly reduced life expectancy – comparable to that of some forms of cancer or triple vessel coronary artery disease.

However, revolutions in understanding the disease processes underlying rheumatoid arthritis, the optimal use of conventional drug therapy and new and exciting developments in drugs, have resulted in a much more optimistic outlook from patients with this disease today and a reduction in the expectation of severe disability that would have been the case, all too often, in the past. This revolution in the management of RA has led to a number of important issues at the interface between primary and secondary care. The nature of the drugs used in rheumatoid arthritis today is such that their careful monitoring may be as important as their administration if therapy is to be safe as well as effective.

Rheumatoid arthritis is a challenging disease, both for sufferers and for those involved in their care. For optimal management of this condition the disease must be diagnosed quickly and appropriate disease-modifying therapy commenced at the earliest opportunity. The multisystem nature of this disease, together with its impact on many activities of daily living, means that a team approach to management of RA is essential. There also is now little doubt that a better understanding of rheumatoid arthritis at all levels, including patients, leads to better outcomes. This book is designed to provide helpful information to all of those involved in the care of patients with rheumatoid arthritis – whether general practitioners, hospital doctors, nurses, therapists or carers. We hope that patients with rheumatoid arthritis may also gain helpful information from this book.

Robert J Moots
Nigel Jones

ACKNOWLEDGEMENTS

We are very grateful to Miss Paula Finnigan for her hard work and patience in preparing this manuscript. We would also like to thank all our colleagues at University Hospital Aintree and Aintree Park Group Practice, Liverpool, UK.

How to use this book

The *Your Questions Answered* series aims to meet the information needs of GPs and other primary care professionals who care for patients with chronic conditions. It is designed to help them work with patients and their families, providing effective, evidence-based care and management.

The books are in an accessible question and answer format, with detailed contents lists at the beginning of every chapter and a complete index to help find specific information.

ICONS
Icons are used in the book to identify particular types of information:

 highlights information important to clinical practice

 highlights side effect information

PATIENT QUESTIONS
At the end of relevant chapters there are sections of frequently asked patient questions, with easy-to-understand answers aimed at the non-medical reader. These questions are also listed at the end of the book.

A background knowledge of rheumatoid arthritis: aetiology, epidemiology and pathology

1

1.1 What is 'arthritis'?

Perhaps surprisingly, arthritis may sometimes be hard to define. For example, as we get older we all are prone to get wrinkles in our skin, which, although perhaps not pleasant, is not a 'disease'. Similarly, as we age we also experience wearing in our joints with loss of cartilage and may have abnormal x-rays as the joints respond by forming new bone to compensate for the wearing. However, when to draw the line between 'wear and tear' and 'osteoarthritis' can be very difficult to determine and is certainly not practical by x-rays, since x-ray changes often do not correlate with pain. What is more important is that people can get severe pain, together with abnormal joint function, which can make a significant impact on life, changing a healthy individual into a 'patient'.

In rheumatoid arthritis (RA) it's much easier to make the distinction between health and disease. In the case of RA, there is a true 'arthritis' with inflammation in a joint resulting in the cardinal signs of inflammation: pain, swelling, redness, heat and loss of function.

1.2 What is 'rheumatism'?

There is no such thing as 'rheumatism' in the strict medical sense. This term is commonly used by people to indicate aches and pains in joints and muscles. It is perceived by many as an almost inevitable consequence of ageing. Therefore, 'rheumatism' or 'rheumatics' tends to be used for conditions which, whilst painful and a nuisance, are not incapacitating to the same extent as 'arthritis'. This pragmatic definition of this term is useful, particularly for older individuals, to distinguish aches and pains from true 'arthritis' – yet still convey the discomfort that is experienced.

1.3 What does 'rheumatoid' mean?

'Rheumatoid' refers to the type of joint disease associated with rheumatoid arthritis. In other words, it refers to joint problems, which are caused by inflammation, result in deformity and destruction of a joint and which untreated can lead to disability. Indeed, 'rheumatoid disease' is actually a much better term than rheumatoid arthritis because, unlike other forms of arthritis, rheumatoid disease (rheumatoid arthritis) can affect any organ of the body and is not purely a disease of the joints.

1.4 What is 'palindromic rheumatism'?

This term refers to one of the various patterns of onset of rheumatoid arthritis. In this situation, people get pain, swelling and stiffness in one or a few joints, which spontaneously resolves. At a later date, which can be weeks, months or occasionally more than a year after the first episode, it is repeated in other joints. The joint inflammation, therefore, 'flits' around the body affecting a few joints, getting better, and then affecting other joints. Usually (but not always) the problem settles down in a rheumatoid joint pattern (see below), evolving into typical rheumatoid arthritis.

It can often be difficult to distinguish palindromic rheumatism (in other words, a palindromic onset of rheumatoid arthritis) from more trivial aches and pains. However, if it is thought to be a clinical possibility, then appropriate tests for potential rheumatoid arthritis should be performed (*see Ch. 3*) as specific therapy might be required.

1.5   How common is rheumatoid arthritis?

Rheumatoid arthritis has an approximate incidence in the UK of 0.5 per 1000 person years. However, with a wide spectrum of disease and many clinical manifestations, some of the milder forms of rheumatoid arthritis might not be recognised and its true incidence may be somewhat higher.

1.6   How prevalent is rheumatoid arthritis?

The prevalence of rheumatoid arthritis in the United Kingdom is more than 1%, making it more common than type I diabetes. Rheumatoid arthritis is perhaps the most common autoimmune disease.

A recent study[1] on the epidemiology and genetics of rheumatoid arthritis charted the prevalence of RA in various populations; this is shown diagrammatically in *Figure. 1.1*.

1.7   Is rheumatoid arthritis hereditary?

There are many factors responsible for the development of rheumatoid arthritis. It is thought to develop by a combination of genetic and environmental factors. There is certainly a hereditary or a genetic link to the development of rheumatoid arthritis; however studies of identical twins[2] have shown that the disease occurs in both of them in only about 30% of cases. The environmental contribution to this disease is therefore greater than the genetic contribution.

When the genetic contribution was assessed in detail, it became apparent that there are a number of genes responsible, rather than just a single gene. However, the gene with the greatest contribution towards genetic susceptibility in rheumatoid arthritis is the major histocompatibility complex (MHC). This gene complex is important in the immune response, and its relationship with RA suggests that the immune system plays an important role in its pathology (and indeed treatment).

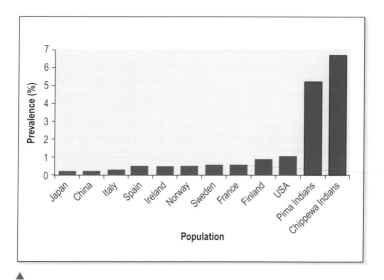

▲

Fig. 1.1 Prevalence of rheumatoid arthritis in various populations. (From Silman & Pearson[1] published by BioMed Central Ltd.)

1.8   Is rheumatoid arthritis more common in men or in women?

Rheumatoid arthritis is more common in women than in men, affecting nearly three women for every man. It is not known why this disease is more common in women, but clearly hormonal differences may play a part. Indeed, when women with rheumatoid arthritis become pregnant they are more likely to enjoy remission of the disease than for the disease to flare-up – highlighting further the likely effect of hormones on this disease.

Furthermore, when rheumatoid arthritis develops in a man the disease may take a more severe course, although this is not a hard and fast rule.

1.9   Is rheumatoid arthritis getting more common?

It is difficult to get high quality data to assess the true incidence of rheumatoid arthritis now compared to formerly, since good detailed epidemiological studies did not occur in the past to the same extent as today to allow for an accurate comparison. However, it is striking that rheumatoid arthritis was never really described in detail until the nineteenth century and, in this respect, rheumatoid arthritis appears to be a 'modern' disease. There certainly appears to have been sporadic cases of rheumatoid arthritis in the past (especially notable in skeletal remains of Pima Indians hundreds of years ago) but corresponding analysis of skeletal remains from other areas over the centuries has not revealed the typical features of rheumatoid arthritis – highlighting the idea that it has tended to occur more recently.

1.10 Are there any racial differences in the incidence of rheumatoid arthritis?

The incidence of rheumatoid arthritis appears to differ more with geographical area than with race. It may be a little less common around Mediterranean areas compared to more northern areas. The reasons underlying these differences are not known. However, a recent report[3] has shown that eating a Mediterranean style diet may relieve symptoms and signs in patients with rheumatoid arthritis.

1.11 What ages does rheumatoid arthritis affect?

Rheumatoid arthritis can develop in people of almost any age. When a disease such as rheumatoid arthritis develops in children it is termed one of the 'juvenile idiopathic arthritides' or JIA. The most common age to develop rheumatoid arthritis is between 40 and 60 but people from teens up until the eighth decade can develop this disease.

1.12 Is rheumatoid arthritis an autoimmune disorder?

The full details of the pathological mechanisms causing rheumatoid arthritis are not yet fully known. There have been many theories proposed to explain the development of rheumatoid arthritis, ranging from exposure to toxins, metabolic problems, through to ongoing infections. However, the balance of evidence points towards an autoimmune aetiology for this disease.

1.13 What does autoimmune mean?

The immune system has evolved to protect us from infection. Inflammation is crucial for infections to resolve. One of the most common causes of synovitis is a viral infection such as influenza or rubella; however the immune system successfully combats the infection and there is resolution of inflammation and improvement in the transient joint aches with these diseases.

In contrast, autoimmune diseases are thought to result from the immune system changing from attacking foreign organisms into attacking self-proteins. The self-proteins that are attacked in rheumatoid arthritis are not known, although it is thought that proteins found within cartilage in synovial joints may be such a target. This has triggered a whole field of research aimed at halting the autoimmune process by either suppressing the immune system or attempting to selectively switch off cells that attack self, by inducing an inhibitory immunological process known as 'tolerance'.

1.14   Is the autoimmune process triggered by a virus?

Exactly what triggers the autoimmune pathological process in rheumatoid arthritis is not yet known. Since the immune system becomes activated by foreign bodies such as viruses, many people believe that, by some mechanism, an infection (possibly a virus) stimulates ('switches on') the immune system appropriately initially. However, in rheumatoid arthritis the immune system does not switch off correctly and as the infection resolves, the immune response changes to become reactive to self-proteins in the joints and the inflammatory process perpetuates, eventually becoming autonomous. Much work is going on at the moment to try to identify how this happens, as blocking it might represent a new way to treat this disease.

1.15   Are there any environmental factors in the causation of rheumatoid arthritis?

Environmental factors probably account for as much as 70% of susceptibility to rheumatoid arthritis. There are many potential factors, which range from infections through lifestyle to diet. Some people have also suggested that the amount of sunlight the body is exposed to can reduce the susceptibility to rheumatoid arthritis to explain the geographical differences. Some studies[4] have shown rheumatoid arthritis is both more prevalent and more severe in areas that are relatively socio-economically deprived. This certainly appears to be the case for the United Kingdom. The reasons underlying this are not fully known.

1.16   Does it matter if people with rheumatoid arthritis smoke?

A number of studies have shown that smoking is linked to rheumatoid arthritis. Some earlier studies suggested that this was only, at best, a weak association. However, more recent work has identified that the cumulative exposure to cigarette smoke, over many years, predisposes some individuals to having a more severe type of rheumatoid arthritis with the presence of rheumatoid nodules and higher disability scores.[5] It has been suggested that active smoking at the onset of rheumatoid disease carries an adverse effect on the progression of the disease, regardless as to whether or not smoking is discontinued. In addition, smoking is associated, in healthy people, with a higher prevalence of rheumatoid factor, an autoantibody found in rheumatoid arthritis.

All available data would suggest that it is advisable to stop smoking in order to reduce the chance of developing rheumatoid arthritis. Once RA has started, however, the benefits of stopping smoking in the disease itself are not known. Since RA carries a higher cardiovascular mortality than in the non-arthritic population, patients with RA who smoke should certainly be advised to stop, in the hope that there will be some reduction in the overall excess cardiovascular mortality.

1.17 What is 'burnt out' rheumatoid arthritis?

'Burnt out' rheumatoid arthritis refers to somebody who has suffered from rheumatoid arthritis in a severe and active form for some (usually considerable) time but in whom there now appears to be no measurable disease activity in their joints. In other words, the joints no longer appear to be swollen with synovitis or shows signs of inflammation – although they certainly are likely to be severely damaged with a whole range of joint deformities. Similarly, blood tests may or may not show signs of inflammation with the raised erythrocyte sedimentation rate (ESR) and C-reactive protein (CRP) found in active rheumatoid arthritis.

Why this disease should appear to resolve spontaneously in these 'burnt out' patients is not yet known. However, treatment for such patients is still required – including supportive measures with occupational therapy, physiotherapy, painkillers and, perhaps, surgery (*see Qs 8.11–8.14*) – rather than an attempt to induce remission with drugs.

1.18 Does rheumatoid arthritis always 'burn out'?

It is more usual for rheumatoid arthritis to run a constant course (albeit with flares and relative remissions during the time) rather than always 'burn out'. Indeed, as patients with rheumatoid arthritis are successfully put into remission by drug therapy it is more usual for the disease to flare up when disease-limiting drugs are removed and, as a consequence, such disease-remitting therapy is usually required lifelong.

1.19 For how long does rheumatoid arthritis run its course?

It is more usual for rheumatoid arthritis to run a constant and progressive course rather than spontaneously remit, although the latter does happen from time to time. It will be interesting to see whether – now that there is a higher alertness to diagnosing and treating this disease very aggressively at the early stage – this will result in the natural history of the disease changing. However, experience to date, even with the best biologic anti-tumour necrosis factor alpha (TNF-alpha) drugs (*see Ch. 7*), suggests that once disease-remitting therapy stops the disease inevitably flares up again.

1.20 What factors are associated with poor prognosis in rheumatoid arthritis?

As yet, there is no ideal way of predicting who is going to do well and who is going to have a very severe and progressive disease course in rheumatoid arthritis. There are a number of helpful factors to consider, the best of which is a simple observation that patients with the worse disease and who are the most incapacitated at the time of diagnosis, tend to suffer the worse disease course! This overall functional activity is assessed by measurement using the disability index of the Health Assessment Questionnaire (HAQ) (*see Appendix 1*), where a poor performance in this instrument determining the patient's function correlates with severe progressive disease in the future. It can also be used to monitor how treatment is improving the patient's life.

Additional factors are also helpful. Patients with rheumatoid arthritis who are rheumatoid factor positive are both more likely to do worse and also to have extra-articular disease. Patients with a particular genetic MHC type (*see Q. 1.7*) of HLA-DR4 or DR1 are also more likely to have a worse disease course.

There is a lot of research underway at present to try and best identify, either clinically or genetically, individuals at risk of the worse disease to allow targeting of the most intensive therapies for these individuals rather than subjecting patients who are likely to have a very mild and perhaps even self-limiting disease to toxic drugs. However, there is still a long way to go before treatment can be best tailored to expected clinical course.

1.21 Is life expectancy reduced in rheumatoid arthritis?

Rheumatoid arthritis is not just a disease of joints, it is a systemic disease, which can kill. Recent studies[6] have shown that rheumatoid arthritis has a significant impact on mortality. Indeed, a middle-aged man developing rheumatoid arthritis can expect a comparable reduction in life expectancy as if he had non-Hodgkin's lymphoma or triple vessel coronary artery disease! This adverse effect on mortality is likely to be reduced by active and aggressive suppression of disease, especially at an early stage.

1.22 What is the cause of death in people with rheumatoid arthritis?

Rheumatoid arthritis is associated with increased mortality in a number of different areas. Patients might develop severe lung disease with a progressive interstitial fibrosing alveolitis, renal impairment, drug toxicity, and many other complicating factors that can lead to death. However, it is emerging that the biggest killer overall in patients with rheumatoid arthritis is an excess cardiovascular mortality. It is therefore important, perhaps more than in many other diseases, to look for cardiovascular risk factors and treat these aggressively in patients with rheumatoid arthritis and, in parallel, suppress the disease activity as much as possible to try to reduce this cardiovascular mortality.

1.23 What are the long term medical and economic consequences of rheumatoid arthritis?

Rheumatoid arthritis has severe long term economic consequences, including direct costs of medical care, indirect costs of work disability and interference with social roles, as well as the intangible costs of pain, fatigue, helplessness, loss of self-efficacy and other psychological difficulties.[7] The consequences of rheumatoid arthritis have often been underestimated. However, new approaches to therapy, including earlier and more aggressive intervention, new drugs and combinations of drugs (*see Chs 5–7 and Appendix 3*), may prevent long term damage and reduce the considerable costs involved.

 PATIENT QUESTIONS

1.24 What has caused my arthritis?

There is no simple answer to this question. There is still very little known about what causes certain people to develop this disease. It is likely to be a combination of the genes which you have inherited from your parents and were born with and exposure to something in the environment, possibly a virus. Arthritis is not, however, 'catching' and cannot be passed from one person to another. There are no particular jobs which make people susceptible to the development of rheumatoid arthritis. Smoking does not cause arthritis, but people who smoke appear to have worse disease compared to those that don't. If you smoke, then this is an extra reason to stop!

1.25 I have rheumatoid arthritis. Will my children get it?

Rheumatoid arthritis, like many other diseases, may run in families. It is not a truly hereditary disease, however, and the children of most people with rheumatoid arthritis never develop any symptoms or signs of this disease. The chances of your children getting rheumatoid arthritis are only very slightly higher than others and the minimal extra risk is too low to cause any real worries.

PATIENT QUESTIONS

1.26   Can my arthritis be cured?

There is no cure for rheumatoid arthritis but it can be fully controlled. It should be remembered that there are now lots of very good drugs available for treating the disease and most patients with rheumatoid arthritis should aim to live a normal life in terms of occupation, family and social activities. Many health care professionals are involved in looking after people with rheumatoid arthritis and there are many places from where you can obtain help or support (*see Appendix 2*).

1.27   Will I end up in a wheelchair?

Treatment for rheumatoid arthritis is long term and depends upon a close and trusting relationship between you and your doctors. Today, it is extremely unlikely that a patient developing rheumatoid arthritis will end up in a wheelchair. However, rheumatoid arthritis is a disease that needs constant treatment with medication and it is important to find the right medication that you can take long term and that will suppress the inflammation in your joints. Stopping medication for reasons other than unacceptable side effects or loss of effectiveness of the drug can result in continued or aggravated inflammation, which, if not suppressed, may damage joints. With a good relationship between you, your general practitioner/primary care physician, and your rheumatology specialist, this does not need to happen.

History and examination

2

2.1 How can I quickly assess whether a patient's joint problem is inflammatory or non-inflammatory?

It is very important to have a quick and easy screening method to try to identify those patients with inflammatory arthritis compared to other forms of arthritis. Inflammatory arthritis is potentially suppressible and considerable disability can be prevented by early detection and treatment. As with most things in medicine, screening for potential inflammatory arthritis depends on history, examination and investigations.

2.2 What are the key questions in the history?

The most important symptom of inflammatory arthritis compared to other joint problems is the presence of profound early morning joint stiffness. Although it is common for many patients with osteoarthritis (and even 'healthy' people) to have a few minutes of joint stiffness on waking, patients with inflammatory arthritis get profound stiffness lasting more than an hour – sometimes all morning or even all day.

In addition to early morning stiffness, patients report stiffness after periods of inactivity, such as sitting down for a while. This is known as 'gelling'.

Rheumatoid arthritis (RA) also causes problems outside the joints and patients with RA often also complain of feeling very 'run down' or are 'exhausted'. The pain and stiffness is typically experienced in hands and feet and patients may say it feels like they are walking on 'broken glass' or 'pebbles' due to metatarsophalangeal (MTP) involvement in their feet. Patients will also report that their joints will feel and look swollen.

2.3 How can I distinguish between rheumatoid arthritis and osteoarthritis?

The main features of patients' symptoms and physical signs in rheumatoid arthritis and osteoarthritis are listed in *Table 2.1*. Sometimes it can be very difficult to distinguish between these two diseases.

The hands are typical places to see changes in many forms of arthritis. *Figure 2.1A* shows the typical changes of osteoarthritis (distal interphalangeal joint involvement and an asymmetrical picture); *Figure 2.1B* shows the typical changes of rheumatoid arthritis (metacarpophalangeal and proximal interphalangeal joint involvement in a symmetrical manner) with typical deformities of ulnar deviation of the digits.

TABLE 2.1 Comparison of major features of rheumatoid arthritis with osteoarthritis (degenerative disease)

Features	Rheumatoid arthritis	Osteoarthritis
Age of onset	All ages	Rare before fifth decade
Sex ratio (female:male)	3:1	Slight female preponderance
Prevalence	0.5–1%	Radiological 50% (> 60 years) Clinical > 10% (> 60 years)
Peak incidence	20–40 years	> 65 years
Systemic features	Yes	No
Joint distribution	Symmetrical (> 75%)	Asymmetrical (> 80%)
Morning stiffness	Marked	Minimal
Synovitis (inflammation)	100%	< 10%
Heberden's (DIP) nodes	No	Yes
Bouchard's (PIP) nodes	No	Yes
Rheumatoid nodules	Yes	No
Rheumatoid factor	Positive in high titre (> 75%)	Positive in low titre (< 5%)
Radiology	Periodic osteoporosis, joint space narrowing, erosions	Osteosclerosis, joint space narrowing, new bone formation, possibly cysts

DIP, distal interphalangeal; PIP, proximal interphalangeal.

2.4 Is rheumatoid arthritis always symmetrical?

Joint involvement in rheumatoid arthritis is typically symmetrical and involves many joints. However, less commonly, other patterns may occur, with only a few joints asymmetrically involved. For example, rheumatoid arthritis may start off with just inflammation in a large joint such as a knee. It may involve a few joints such as the left wrist, right hand, and right ankle – or just a few knuckles.

In elderly patients, the onset of rheumatoid arthritis may be very difficult to distinguish from polymyalgia rheumatica. This is termed the 'polymyalgic' onset of rheumatoid arthritis. The fact that these patients may be given steroids on the assumption that polymyalgia rheumatica may mask symptoms of rheumatoid arthritis makes the true diagnosis of RA much harder to determine.

2.5 In which joints is rheumatoid arthritis commonest?

Rheumatoid arthritis tends to affect small joints – many at a time. Hands, wrists and feet are particularly involved. However, other synovial joints –

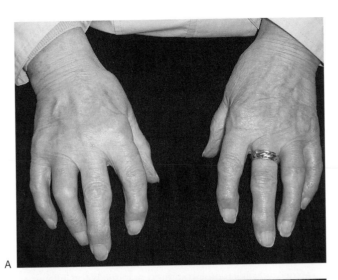

A

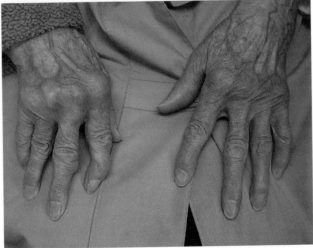

B

Fig. 2.1 A, Typical changes of osteoarthritis with a symmetrical involvement and particular involvement of distal and interphalangeal joints; **B**, typical changes of rheumatoid arthritis with a symmetrical involvement, ulnar deviation of fingers and a more proximal interphalangeal joint and metacarpophalangeal joint involvement.

particularly shoulders, wrists, knees and neck – are also often involved. Rheumatoid arthritis also affects temporomandibular joints, ankles and elbows. The distribution of joints affected in RA is illustrated in *Figure 2.2*.

Rheumatoid arthritis does not affect non-synovial joints and is not responsible for low back pain for example.

2.6 What is a 'typical rheumatoid distribution'?

Rheumatoid arthritis typically affects many small joints, on both sides of the body – a symmetrical, small joint polyarthritis. The small joints in the hands and feet are particularly involved. Within the hands, the metacarpophalangeal (MCP) and proximal interphalangeal (PIP) joints are affected – but not the distal interphalangeal (DIP) joints.

In contrast, osteoarthritis (OA) tends to affect a few joints – especially larger ones such as hips and knees. When OA affects the small joints of the hand, it is usually the base of the thumb or DIP joints and is easily recognised. However, OA of the hands can sometimes be confused with RA – but in OA there is not the associated early morning stiffness or raised blood inflammatory markers as found in RA.

2.7 What is 'synovitis'?

The term 'synovitis' means inflammation of the synovial membrane. This membrane lines synovial joints, such as those found in the hands, feet, shoulders, elbows, wrists, hips, neck and knees. As synovitis progresses there is swelling of affected joints. Such swelling is caused by a combination of increased joint fluid and proliferating synovial tissue, which changes from a very delicate membrane surrounding the joint to a tumour-like cauliflower structure known as a pannus.

On examination, a joint with synovitis will be swollen and tender, it will feel fluctuant with an excess of synovial fluid and have a 'boggy' swelling due to proliferation of synovial tissue. The joint will be warm and tend to have a reduced range of movement. Synovitis is most easily detected in large joints such as the knee, in the wrist and in the knuckles (MCP and PIP joints).

2.8 How do I check for synovitis?

Synovitis in the hands can often be detected simply by offering to shake hands with a patient, who will try to avoid this because of the pain. In addition, knuckles and PIP joints will be swollen. Synovitis in knees can be detected by gentle palpation of the joint, feeling fluctuance, and often

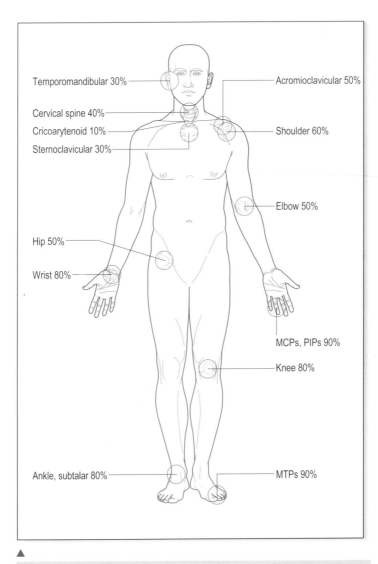

Fig. 2.2 Joint distribution of rheumatoid arthritis. MCPs, metacarpophalangeal joints; PIPs, proximal interphalangeal joints.

demonstrating a 'patellar tap' where gentle pressure on a patella with a patient lying flat on their back will result in a patella moving down to press on the tibia. Normally the patella is in close contact with a tibia and cannot be 'tapped' on to it; in RA swollen joints, the extra synovial fluid presses the patella up and away from the tibia. However, where there is a large proliferation of synovial tissue, rather than fluid in a joint, a patellar tap may be absent, even if the joint is obviously very swollen.

2.9 What extra-articular symptoms are common in rheumatoid arthritis?

Although called 'rheumatoid arthritis', RA might better be termed 'rheumatoid disease', since it does not only affect joints. Indeed, pretty well any organ in the body can be involved to some extent by this disease!

One of the most common extra-articular symptoms is that of fatigue, which mirrors the profound inflammatory response. However, as the disease progresses, patients may complain of a number of problems (*see Fig. 2.3*) including:

- lumps and bumps (rheumatoid nodules) around tendons, especially elbows, which are more common in seropositive patients and in smokers
- symptoms related to the anaemia of chronic disease
- leg ulcers (vasculitis).

2.10 What are the rare extra-articular complications of rheumatoid arthritis?

In addition to the problems outlined above, patients with rheumatoid arthritis at later stages of disease may develop splinter haemorrhages and nailfold infarcts. There can be pleural effusions, pericarditis, conducting system abnormalities in the heart, splenomegaly, neutropenia, amyloidosis neuropathy, interstitial lung disease, and many other rare features. All extra-articular manifestations of disease in RA tend to occur in patients with severe longstanding seropositive (rheumatoid factor positive) disease – good control of RA may reduce the frequency of these complications. Extra-articular rheumatoid disease is summarised in *Box 2.1*.

2.11 What is the GALS assessment?

GALS stands for Gait, Arms, Legs, Spine. It is a well recognised musculoskeletal screening routine which, once learnt, can aid rapid assessment of musculoskeletal problems in the general practice/primary care setting. It is most easily performed by the doctor undertaking the movements and asking the patient to copy.

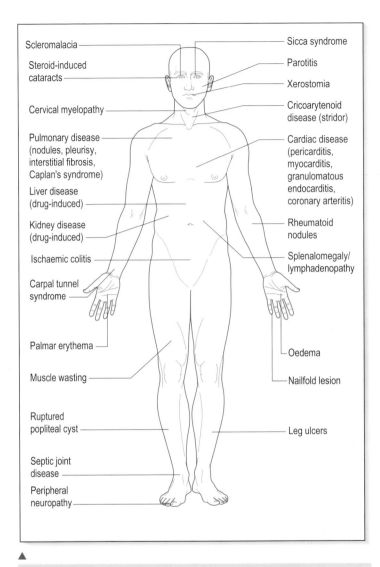

Fig. 2.3 Common extra-articular symptoms and signs in rheumatoid disease.

BOX 2.1 Extra-articular manifestations of rheumatoid arthritis

- Rheumatoid nodules
- Vasculitis
- Pulmonary
  — pleural effusion
  — fibrosing alveolitis
  — nodules
- Cardiac
  — pericarditis
  — mitral valve disease
  — conduction defects
- Skin
  — palmar erythema
  — cutaneous vasculitis
  — pyoderma gangrenosum
  — ulcers

GAIT

- Observe the patient walking, turning and walking back, looking for smoothness and symmetry of limb and pelvic movements, normal stride length and the ability to turn quickly.

ARMS

- Inspect from the front, assessing muscle bulk and symmetry.
- With both hands down by the sides and the elbows fully extended, the patient should attempt to place both hands behind their head and then push the elbows back; assess glenohumeral, acromioclavicular and sternoclavicular joint function.
- Examine the hands with palms down and fingers straight. Look for swelling or deformity.
- Observe normal pronation/supination and grip.
- Ask the patient to place the tip of each finger onto the tip of the thumb in turn to assess normal dexterity and fine precision pinch.
- Squeeze across the patient's second to fifth metacarpals (pain suggests synovitis).

LEGS

- Inspect the patient standing. Look for any knee or foot deformity.
- On the examination couch, look for and test for knee effusion (patellar tap).

- Test flexion of each hip and knee. When doing this, have your hand on the patient's knee to assess crepitus.
- Check passive internal rotation of each hip.
- Squeeze across the metatarsals to detect synovitis.
- Inspect the soles of the feet noting any callosities or rashes

SPINE
- From behind, is the spine straight?
- Are the iliac crests level and is paraspinal muscle bulk equal both sides?
- Assess lateral cervical spine flexion by asking the patient to place their ear on their shoulder.
- From the side, again note any spinal curvature.
- Ask the patient to bend forward and touch their toes with their knees straight; assess function of lumbar spine and hip flexion.

2.12 How useful is the GALS?

The GALS is a helpful rapid screening tool to pick up significant joint problems. It can be performed very quickly and easily and can help identify problems that can be investigated further by a more detailed history and examination.

2.13 What are rheumatoid nodules?

Rheumatoid nodules are soft tissue nodular lumps, which are found only in patients with rheumatoid arthritis, and then only in those who have rheumatoid factor (in other words, seropositive RA). Histologically, rheumatoid nodules are made up of chronic inflammatory cells and fibrotic cells. This is one situation where an antibody (rheumatoid factor) can be detected by clinical examination alone, without the need for a blood test. Whilst only patients who are seropositive for rheumatoid factor can get rheumatoid nodules, only about a third of patients with seropositive rheumatoid arthritis may suffer from nodules.

2.14 Where do these nodules occur?

Rheumatoid nodules can occur in almost any part of the body, externally or internally. Externally they are prone to occur at sites of shearing stress, most typically around the extensor side of the elbow and forearm, together with pressure points around the feet, buttocks and hands. At these areas the rheumatoid nodules are usually subcutaneous but may sometimes be subperiosteal. Internally, they may occur in the lungs, where they can be mistaken for metastatic carcinoma, but can rarely appear in the heart, where they may cause conduction disturbances, in the larynx, where they may cause speech problems, or indeed in other internal structures.

2.15 How is a diagnosis of rheumatoid arthritis formally made?

Rheumatoid arthritis is diagnosed according to the 1987 revised criteria by the American Rheumatism Association (now the American College of Rheumatology, ACR). These criteria are listed in *Box 2.2*.

2.16 How relevant are the ACR criteria?

It is important that rheumatoid arthritis is diagnosed correctly, in order to institute appropriate treatment. The 1987 ACR criteria were a major advance in helping to classify and understand rheumatoid arthritis. However, these criteria are not perfect. It is now known that joint damage can occur as early as 3 months into the disease. It is certainly unfortunate that the original ACR criteria required patients to have symptoms for some months to qualify formally for a diagnosis of rheumatoid arthritis because this would delay appropriate treatment and result in early, potentially avoidable, joint damage. It is therefore inappropriate to wait before considering a diagnosis of rheumatoid arthritis.

2.17 What are the more unusual presentations of rheumatoid arthritis?

Apart from the typical symmetrical small joint polyarthritis, rheumatoid arthritis can present in other ways:

- There may be just one or two joints involved at the start.
- Extra-articular features such as nodules may develop rarely ahead of joint problems.
- A few joints may become involved, get better, and then a different group of joints become involved (palindromic onset).
- Fatigue and anaemia of chronic disease may precede overt joint involvement.

2.18 Can rheumatoid arthritis present as anything other than a joint problem?

It is very rare for RA to start without significant joint problems. However, RA can sometimes present with fatigue, anaemia of chronic disease, nodules, or other extra-articular involvement before joints get involved.

2.19 How common are respiratory symptoms/signs in rheumatoid arthritis?

Respiratory system involvement is emerging as a more common extra-articular feature of RA than was previously thought. In early disease this is

---

BOX 2.2 The American College of Rheumatology revised criteria for rheumatoid arthritis classification

1. **Morning stiffness**: lasting 1 hour or more before maximal improvement.

2. **Arthritis in 3 or more joint areas**: at least 3 joint areas simultaneously have soft tissue swelling or fluid (not bony overgrowth alone). The 14 possible areas are: right or left PIP, MCP, wrist, elbow, knee, ankle and MTP joints.

3. **Arthritis of hand joints**: at least 1 area swollen (as defined above) in a wrist, MCP or PIP joint.

4. **Symmetrical arthritis**: simultaneous involvement of the same joint areas (as defined above) on both sides of the body (bilateral involvement of PIPs, MCPs, or MTPs without absolute symmetry is acceptable).

5. **Presence of rheumatoid nodules**: subcutaneous nodules over bony prominences or extensor surfaces or in juxta-articular regions, as observed by a physician.

6. **Positive rheumatoid factor**: demonstration of abnormal amounts of serum rheumatoid factor by a method for which the result has been positive in < 5% of normal control subjects.

7. **Radiographic changes**: radiological changes typical of rheumatoid arthritis on posteroanterior hand and wrist radiographs, which must include erosions or unequivocal bony decalcification localised in or most marked adjacent to the involved joint (osteoarthritic changes alone do not qualify).

For classification purposes, a patient shall be said to have rheumatoid arthritis if they satisfy at least 4 of these 7 criteria. Criteria 1–4 must have been present for at least 6 weeks. Patients with two clinical diagnoses are not excluded.

---

rarely a problem. However, in patients with longstanding disease it may become a major problem. Although rheumatoid arthritis is associated with a higher prevalence of bronchiectasis, the reasons underlying this association are not yet clear. Whilst bronchiectasis may be symptomatic, it may sometimes only be detected on detailed investigations by CT scan.

Interstitial inflammatory lung disease, leading to fibrosis, is also common. Again, this may be asymptomatic, or obvious clinically with, for example, breathlessness and inspiratory crackles – however by this stage it may be too late to treat. It appears that many patients with established rheumatoid arthritis have significant interstitial lung disease which may be asymptomatic. Whether aggressive investigation in asymptomatic patients is indicated and early cytotoxic therapy instituted, is currently under debate.

2.20 What is Felty's syndrome?

Felty's syndrome occurs when patients with seropositive rheumatoid arthritis develop hypersplenism with neutropenia. Associated with this may be increased propensity to infection, skin rash or ulcers. Patients with Felty's syndrome may have a 'burnt out' appearance of rheumatoid arthritis in their joints (i.e. little evidence for active synovitis); however, there is still profound systemic inflammation. The occurrence of Felty's syndrome today seems to be considerably less than in the past. It is now seen only rarely but can be a very worrying and difficult to manage complication of rheumatoid arthritis.

2.21 When should I refer a patient with suspected rheumatoid arthritis to a rheumatologist?

As a serious multisystem inflammatory disease that is associated with profound morbidity and mortality, all patients with rheumatoid arthritis should be seen and assessed by a rheumatologist. Whether long term therapy should be provided by a rheumatologist alone, shared between a rheumatologist and a primary care physician or in primary care alone will depend upon the initial assessment by a rheumatologist and, of course, local experience, expertise and facilities.

It has now been clearly shown that rheumatic disease progress can best be modified and disability minimised, if treated early. It is therefore essential to refer patients with suspected rheumatoid arthritis to a rheumatologist at the earliest opportunity, where there is the maximal chance for successful intervention and disease suppression (*see also Q.10.5*).

PATIENT QUESTIONS

2.22   Why do my joints swell up?

In rheumatoid arthritis joints become inflamed: '-itis' at the end of a word means inflammation. Swelling, along with pain, redness and heat are the well-known signs of inflammation. The swelling is caused by inflammation in your joints, which produces an excess of joint lubricating fluid and overgrowth of soft tissues within your joints.

2.23   Why do I feel so tired?

Having rheumatoid arthritis does not just affect your joints. Tiredness ('feeling run down') is very common in rheumatoid arthritis and is one of the body's natural reactions to many diseases. Our white blood cells form part of our 'immune system', which helps protect us from infections. When this system is asked by our body to work hard – for example when fighting infection or, in the case of rheumatoid arthritis, causing inflammation – we often feel very tired.

2.24   What are these lumps on my skin?

The lumps on your skin are called rheumatoid nodules and are another sign of the inflammation that is occurring throughout your body. These lumps may not look good and may sometimes hurt if they are knocked, but they are not dangerous and are nothing to do with other types of lumps, such as those that may be caused by cancers.

   These nodules do not require any treatment and can safely be left alone. However, if they are unsightly, or prone to hurt when they get knocked, they can be shrunk down by steroid injection or sometimes cut out by surgery. It should be borne in mind, however, that if they have been surgically removed, they may grow back again.

Laboratory tests in rheumatoid arthritis

3

3.1 What simple haematological and biochemical blood tests should I be doing in primary care when rheumatoid arthritis is suspected?

> The most important tests to do are erythrocyte sedimentation rate (ESR) and C-reactive protein (CRP). Additional tests which can be useful, although less so than the above, are a full blood count (FBC) and rheumatoid factor.

3.2 What am I looking for in the results?

The most important blood tests in diagnosing rheumatoid arthritis (RA) are those that measure inflammation. A significantly elevated ESR or CRP suggests inflammation and, with an appropriate clinical picture, inflammatory arthritis. In a FBC, there may be the anaemia of chronic disease associated with rheumatoid arthritis. Such anaemia, whilst more often than not occurring relatively late, can certainly be present at diagnosis and would be entirely in keeping with RA. In addition, a raised platelet count, which corresponds with the inflammatory process, may be often detected. If the patient is taking aspirin or other non-steroidal anti-inflammatory drugs (NSAIDs) there may obviously be a low mean corpuscular volume (MCV) due to iron deficiency anaemia.

3.3 What is ESR?

ESR stands for erythrocyte sedimentation rate. It is a cheap and simple non-specific test for general inflammation, which measures the rate at which red blood cells in a thin column settle over a period of 1 hour, expressed as mm/hr. The more inflammation that is present, the less the forces of repulsion between individual red cells and the faster the column settles. It becomes significant in a young person when it is above 30 mm/hr. However, many older people run a slightly elevated ESR (below 40) without any obvious disease.

   Apart from inflammation, the ESR can also be raised in anaemia and of course in cancers, especially multiple myeloma. The ESR is a good test for screening for inflammation but tends to change relatively slowly as inflammation comes and goes. In active RA, the ESR may rise above 100 mm/hr!

3.4 What is plasma viscosity?

This is a blood test that measures crudely the viscosity of blood, which may correlate with inflammation. This is becoming much less widely used in the

United Kingdom. It is an indirect marker of inflammation that is less effective than ESR and CRP.

3.5 What is CRP?

C-reactive protein (CRP) is an acute phase protein. This is synthesised in the liver in response to proinflammatory cytokines such as interleukin 6 (IL-6) which are secreted as part of the inflammatory response – in the case of RA, produced in inflamed joints. The CRP therefore becomes elevated in inflammation. CRP concentrations in the blood change much quicker than does the ESR, as the inflammatory process waxes and wanes. This test is, therefore, more useful than the ESR in assessing changes in inflammation, such as in response to therapy, where the concentration of CRP may fall as inflammation is suppressed, whereas the ESR will drop much more slowly.

It is often useful to perform an ESR and CRP test in parallel. In RA, the CRP may also rise above 100. In some conditions, such as systemic lupus erythematosus (SLE), the inflammatory response typically results in a high ESR but normal CRP. Similarly, anaemia can result in an elevated ESR but normal CRP. In active RA, the CRP is only exceptionally normal and is almost always elevated.

3.6 What are autoantibodies?

Autoantibodies are antibodies that react against self-proteins rather than foreign viruses and bacteria. Antibodies directed against self-proteins are not necessarily pathological in their own right. Some exist normally, as part of the body's mechanism to control inflammation and repair tissues, helping in general cellular and organ housekeeping activities. However, some autoantibodies, when present in relatively high amounts, are associated with disease.

Perhaps the most common autoantibody is rheumatoid factor (see below). Other autoantibodies that are often found in rheumatoid arthritis include anti-nuclear factor or anti-single stranded DNA antibodies. However, their significance is much less than that of rheumatoid factor.

3.7 What is anti-nuclear antibody?

Anti-nuclear antibodies (ANA) – sometimes known as anti-nuclear factors (ANF) – are a group of autoantibodies that react against components from the nuclei of cells. They are relatively non-specific antibodies with respect to individual disease associations. However, when more of these antibodies are present in correspondingly higher titres, they become more significant. Anti-nuclear antibodies are associated with a variety of autoimmune diseases such as systemic lupus erythematosus, scleroderma and other connective tissue diseases rather than RA (*Box 3.1*). However, they may be useful in detecting complications of treatment such as the development of lupus when taking the antibiotic minocycline (*see Qs 7.1–7.3*).

3.8 What is rheumatoid factor?

Rheumatoid factors are antibodies, which react with a part of other antibodies – the Fc portion of immunoglobulin G (IgG) (*see Fig. 3.1*). Rheumatoid factors can be of any class (or type) of immunoglobulin but the standard tests are designed to detect immunoglobulin M (IgM) rheumatoid factors. Patients with a clinical diagnosis of rheumatoid arthritis may be seropositive or seronegative according to the presence of rheumatoid factors in their blood.

3.9 What blood tests measure rheumatoid factors?

The tests most widely used to measure rheumatoid factors are the rheumatoid latex agglutination (rheumatoid latex) and red cell agglutination tests. In both of these tests, IgG is bound to the surface of particles, which may be latex beads or red cells, and mixed with serum from patients. If rheumatoid factors are present, the factors cause agglutination of the particles to give a positive result. The results are therefore either positive, where agglutination occurs, or negative. If the test is positive then the serum may be diluted further to give a titred result. A cut-off point for a positive result varies between different test systems and laboratories. The type of immunoglobulin used varies with the test. On the whole, the latex

---

BOX 3.1 Conditions in which anti-nuclear antibodies are found

- Systemic lupus erythematosus – approximately 95%
- Sjögren's syndrome – approximately 75%
- Scleroderma – 25%
- Inflammatory muscle disease (polymyositis and dermatomyositis) – 75% (in low titre)
- Rheumatoid arthritis – 30%
- Chronic infections (such as tuberculosis)
- Chronic active hepatitis
- Malignancies
- Healthy people (in low titre of < 1/80)

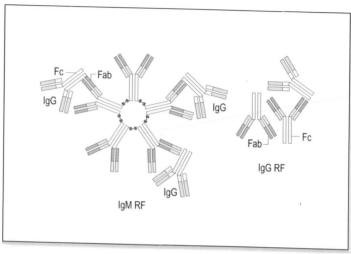

Fig. 3.1 Chemical structure of rheumatoid factor. Fab, antigen binding portion of the antibody; Fc, constant (non-antigen binding) portion of the antibody; IgG RF, immunoglobulin G rheumatoid factor; IgM RF, immunoglobulin M rheumatoid factor.

test uses human immunoglobulin whereas the red cell test (Rose-Waaler) uses rabbit immunoglobulin.

3.10 Can rheumatoid factor be present in the serum of 'normal' people?

Approximately 1 in 20 (5%) of normal healthy people have measurable rheumatoid factor. Furthermore, in otherwise healthy people who smoke quite heavily, there is an even higher association with rheumatoid factor. It is therefore not diagnostic for rheumatoid arthritis but, as below, can be helpful in establishing the prognosis of an individual who has been diagnosed to have RA.

3.11 How often is rheumatoid factor absent in the serum of people with rheumatoid arthritis?

Approximately one-third of patients with rheumatoid arthritis lack rheumatoid factor. These patients are described as being 'seronegative'. On the whole, patients with seronegative rheumatoid arthritis have a slightly better chance of following a more benign course than patients with seropositive RA. They are also much less likely to get extra-articular disease and do not get rheumatoid nodules.

3.12 Is the presence of rheumatoid factor in serum age related?

There is a trend towards the detection of rheumatoid factor with advancing age in otherwise healthy people. Therefore, a strongly positive rheumatoid factor in a young person may be more significant than a corresponding result in an older person.

3.13 When is a rheumatoid factor titre level significant?

If the RA latex test is a general screening for significant autoantibodies, then the rheumatoid factor titre level is a more clinically relevant test (performed in parallel in most laboratories when the RA latex test is positive). The higher the rheumatoid factor titre, the more likely the test is to be significant. It is not possible to give an absolute cut-off point for when this test becomes significant or not, since rheumatoid factor does not diagnose rheumatoid arthritis. However, as the rheumatoid factor titre increases into the hundreds or especially into the thousands, it is much more likely that a patient will have rheumatoid arthritis.

3.14 How high can rheumatoid factor titre levels get?

Rheumatoid factor titres can get into the tens of thousands and at this amount tends to become very significant (although still not diagnostic).

3.15 Is the rheumatoid factor titre level proportional to severity of disease?

There is no hard and fast rule with regard to the rheumatoid factor titre and the severity of disease. As a rule of thumb, however, patients with rheumatoid arthritis and very strongly positive titres of rheumatoid factor are more likely to have severe disease and more likely to have extra-articular disease complications.

3.16 With what other chronic conditions is rheumatoid factor associated?

Rheumatoid factor can be associated both with health and with chronic disease such as other connective tissue diseases (e.g. systemic lupus erythematosus) and chronic infections (e.g. infective endocarditis), as well as chronic obstructive pulmonary disease and bronchiectasis – possibly because smoking is linked to these two diseases and also with the development of rheumatoid factor. Conditions in which rheumatoid factor is found are summarised in *Box 3.2*.

3.17 Are there any other autoantibodies important in rheumatoid arthritis?

A whole variety of autoantibodies apart from rheumatoid factor can often be detected in rheumatoid arthritis. Anti-nuclear factor and anti-single stranded DNA antibodies are two examples. However, these antibodies are less helpful than rheumatoid factor in confirming a diagnosis and also do not correlate with disease severity or progression.

3.18 How is disease activity measured in a rheumatology clinic?

In a rheumatology clinic and especially in trials of anti-rheumatic drugs, it is important to have an objective marker for disease activity to allow any significant change in the patient's condition to be detected. Two important tools are the disease activity score (DAS) 28 and the American College of Rheumatology (ACR) response criteria:

- The DAS 28 is a composite score comprising clinical measures of disease activity (tender joints, swollen joints, patient's global assessment of disease) and an objective laboratory marker, the ESR.[1] This score gives an absolute measure of disease activity. A score of greater than 5.1 indicates severe disease and is one of the current prerequisites for institution of biologic therapy in the UK.
- The ACR response criteria are useful to determine changes in disease activity.[2,3] As with the DAS 28 score, this is a composite figure based on clinical and laboratory variables. There are three main scores – the

---

BOX 3.2 Conditions in which rheumatoid factor is found

- Rheumatoid arthritis – 70%
- Sjögren's syndrome – 50–60%
- Systemic lupus erythematosus – 20%
- Sarcoidosis
- Systemic vasculitis
- Multiple myeloma (and other malignancies)
- Chronic infections (infective endocarditis, leprosy, syphilis, and up to 40% of tuberculosis)
- Chronic liver disease
- Healthy people

ACR 20, 50 and 70. These correspond to an overall improvement of 20% through to 70% in the patient's disease. An ACR 20 is not particularly significant whereas an ACR 70 implies a major reduction in disease activity.

3.19 What is the HAQ?

The Health Assessment Questionnaire (HAQ) is a self-administered, patient completed, questionnaire (*see Appendix 1*). The disability index of this instrument provides a series of questions to patients about their function, in as much as what they can and cannot do, and also what additional aids they need to be able to complete certain tasks. It is a very useful tool, which has been fully validated in rheumatoid arthritis, and the score from the questionnaire can be used to monitor how patients are coping with their arthritis and responding to treatment.

A recent review of the HAQ – its history, issues, progress and documentation – can be found in Bruce & Fries.[4]

3.20 What blood tests should I do in a patient with established disease and why?

Once rheumatoid arthritis has become established it is important to check blood tests from time to time to monitor response to treatment and safety, where disease-modifying drugs are used, and also to investigate for potential complications of this disease. As the disease progresses, for example, it is not unusual to develop the anaemia of chronic disorder. Similarly, the onset of the nowadays rarely seen Felty's syndrome (*see Q. 2.20*) with hypersplenism might result in profound neutropenias. Intercurrent infections and other such problems may also affect the FBC and renal involvement with systemic rheumatoid vasculitis may of course affect renal function tests. Therefore, any patient with established rheumatoid arthritis who becomes ill may require blood tests to help elucidate the cause of the deterioration or detect intercurrent illness.

PATIENT QUESTIONS

3.21 If arthritis affects joints, why am I having blood tests as well as x-rays?

Rheumatoid arthritis is often very difficult to detect with an x-ray until the disease is well established. As well as listening carefully to your story and examining you thoroughly, your doctor can look for certain things in your blood which become raised when you have inflammation in your joints. This can help the doctor make an accurate diagnosis of your problem and start or alter your treatment to offer you the greatest help. As well as helping your doctor make the diagnosis of rheumatoid arthritis, blood tests can help your doctor in assessing how well your disease is responding to treatment. Good doctors will, however, always treat the patient and not the blood test results!

3.22 My blood tests show I have got rheumatoid factor. Does that mean I have rheumatoid arthritis?

Your doctor has checked your blood tests because you have sore joints. Rheumatoid factor is an antibody which is present in approximately two out of three people with rheumatoid arthritis. However, this antibody is also present in at least 1 in 20 normal healthy people. This is a helpful blood test for your doctor but does not make a diagnosis of rheumatoid arthritis. Your doctor will look at other blood tests and see how they fit with what is found when you are physically examined before any diagnosis is made. If your blood tests otherwise are fine and there is no evidence of inflammation in your joints, your doctor will be able to reassure you that you are just one of the many healthy people that have this antibody without any harm at all. However, if there is any uncertainty as to whether you have rheumatoid arthritis or not, or if your tests definitely suggest that rheumatoid arthritis is present, your doctor will refer you on to a rheumatologist who will double check the diagnosis and provide help for you.

Confirming the diagnosis – what's RA and what's not

4.1 What are the other symmetrical inflammatory arthropathies?

Rheumatoid arthritis (RA) is the typical example of a symmetrical inflammatory arthropathy, although there are a number of other conditions which can bear many similarities to RA and be confused with it. These are listed in *Box 4.1*. Psoriatic arthritis in particular can have an indistinguishable pattern of joint involvement from rheumatoid arthritis. In addition to this pattern, psoriatic arthritis can also exhibit other joint involvement patterns ranging from an arthritis mutilans (where there is a rapid destruction of joints of the hands to leave totally functionless 'mutilated' hands) through an ankylosing spondylitis-type picture (with sacroiliitis and early morning stiffness in the lower back – spreading upwards with time) to an oligoarthritis and an inflammatory process affecting the distal interphalangeal joints alone (which may sometimes be confused with the Heberden's nodes of primary nodal osteoarthritis).

Perhaps the most likely cause for at least a transient peripheral inflammatory arthropathy is that of a reaction to a viral infection. This is usually easy to spot as it is less severe and tends to get better very quickly. Many different viruses can cause this. These range from influenza through measles to rubella and parvovirus.

4.2 How can I discount such arthropathies quickly with history/examination?

It is very important to identify that the patient has an inflammatory arthropathy, because this requires urgent referral to a consultant rheumatologist. As such, the presence of synovitis, together with early morning joint stiffness and a raised erythrocyte sedimentation rate (ESR) and/or C-reactive protein (CRP) are paramount. Other forms of inflammatory arthropathy (e.g. psoriatic arthritis) also need referral to a rheumatologist and will equally require disease-modifying therapy – and at an early stage, if damage is to be prevented.

Other confusing patterns of joint involvement, such as primary nodal osteoarthritis which can affect small joints of the hand, can usually be discounted by the clinical picture (distal interphalangeal joint involvement in osteoarthritis versus metacarpophalangeal and proximal interphalangeal joint involvement in rheumatoid arthritis; *see Fig. 2.1*) together with normal inflammatory markers in osteoarthritis. However, it is sometimes very difficult to distinguish between these two totally different diseases in the early stages.

> **BOX 4.1 Conditions that may be confused with rheumatoid arthritis**
>
> ■ Connective tissue disease (especially systemic lupus erythematosus)
> ■ Psoriatic arthritis
> ■ Polymyalgia rheumatica
> ■ Inflammatory osteoarthritis
> ■ Seronegative spondyloarthropathy
> ■ Gout (polyarticular)
> ■ Pseudogout
> ■ Multicentric reticulohistiocytosis
> ■ Sickle cell disease

4.3 Can rheumatoid arthritis be clinically quantified?

Counting the number of swollen joints from which a patient is suffering and measuring the degree of joint tenderness can be useful in clinically monitoring rheumatoid arthritis. The correlation between joint swelling and tenderness is quite poor, which is why both need to be assessed.

There is as yet no consensus on a single standardised method of assessing RA. The methods available vary in the number of joints assessed, whether these joints are weighted according to size (large versus small) and whether the joint abnormality is scored on a linear scale or simply as being normal or abnormal:

■ A joint count is obtained when the number of abnormal joints is recorded.
■ A joint score is obtained when the abnormality is graded and/or weighted.
■ Joint counts may be more reproducible than joint scores.

The 'Ritchie articular index', which has been widely used in the UK, is an example of a tender joint score. Fifty-two peripheral joints or joint areas are graded on a 4-point scale for tenderness. Similarly, the DAS 28 score (*see Q. 3.18*) gives an absolute value as to the amount of disease activity in rheumatoid arthritis whereas the American College of Rheumatology (ACR) response criteria can be useful in assessing the degree of improvement but not absolute activity.

4.4 Are x-rays helpful in diagnosing rheumatoid arthritis?

X-rays are very useful in following the longer term course of rheumatoid arthritis but are not helpful in making an early diagnosis. It should be remembered that radiological investigations are only of value if they are going to alter the management of the patient. Is there something that we can see on an x-ray that would make us change our mind in terms of diagnosis or treatment? If the decision to perform an x-ray is purely to satisfy the patient or for academic interest then the test may be better avoided in primary care.

The cardinal features of joint involvement in rheumatoid arthritis on x-ray are joint space narrowing, peri-articular osteoporosis, soft tissue shadowing around joints and erosions. The only really discriminating x-ray appearance is that of erosions (*see Fig. 4.1*); these happen relatively late and indicate that irreversible damage has already occurred. The ideal thing is to prevent the development of erosions and this really means treatment within the first 3–6 months of onset of disease.

4.5 Which joints should be x-rayed?

The most sensitive joints in which to detect involvement of rheumatoid arthritis are those in the hands and feet. As the disease progresses and if not amenable to disease-suppressing therapy, then x-ray appearances can develop in other synovial joints (e.g. large joints such as the hip and knee) and the cervical spine. Rheumatoid arthritis does not affect the lumbosacral spine or the sacroiliac joints and is not a cause of low back pain.

X-rays are also obviously required when planning surgery or when assessing for anaesthesia a patient with severe neck pain to make sure that standard intubation techniques are safe and that there is no risk of transecting the spinal cord from an unstable neck. Such instability will require urgent magnetic resonance imaging and, potentially, referral of the patient by the rheumatologist to a neurosurgeon.

In general, serial x-ray films are of limited benefit but may have a minor role to play in the occasional patient with rheumatoid arthritis when there is uncertainty about disease progression.

4.6 What are erosions?

Erosions are small areas of focal bone loss at the edge of joints. The x-ray appearance is that of a mouse bite nibbling the edge of a joint (*Fig. 4.1*) and is an indicator of bone and joint destruction. Erosions at joint margins are typical features of rheumatoid arthritis and show that significant joint damage has already occurred.

4.7 How common are erosions in rheumatoid arthritis?

Unfortunately, erosions have until recently been inevitable in patients with rheumatoid arthritis. Only patients running a particularly benign disease

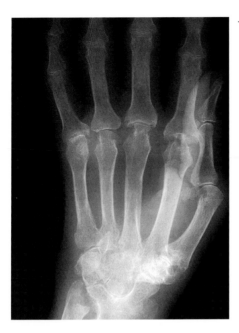

◀ **Fig. 4.1** Radiograph of a hand of a patient with rheumatoid arthritis showing periarticular osteoporosis, some joint space narrowing and erosions around the joint margin of metacarpophalangeal joints.

course would escape without the development of erosions and even then, the diagnosis of RA would be under doubt. In the past, the diagnosis of rheumatoid arthritis was confirmed only by the development of erosions. The aim of specialist therapy for rheumatoid arthritis today, however, is to prevent the development of erosions and subsequent joint damage. Despite everyone's best efforts, however, even those patients who are diagnosed early and undergo rapid aggressive therapy often go on to develop radiological evidence of joint erosions.

4.8 Is it always easy to diagnose rheumatoid arthritis?

A typical 'barn door' presentation of rheumatoid arthritis is very easy. However, some patients develop rheumatoid arthritis very slowly and with few symptoms. In these circumstances, it is often useful to keep a relatively open mind with such patients and check them over from time to time both clinically and with blood tests until the situation becomes clear. However, once there is a reasonable index of suspicion for an inflammatory process it is mandatory to refer patients to a rheumatologist.

One study[1] on the articular patterns in the early course of rheumatoid arthritis demonstrated a monocyclic pattern (single cycle with remission for at least 1 year) in 20% of cases, a progressive pattern (increasing joint involvement) in 10% of cases and a polycyclic pattern (patients with either intermittent or continuous subtypes) in 70% of cases (*Fig. 4.2*).

4.9 What should I do as a GP if I'm unsure as to whether or not a patient has rheumatoid arthritis?

Sometimes it can be hard to diagnose rheumatoid arthritis if it presents in an unusual manner or comes on slowly. When there is clinical uncertainty, elevated blood tests for inflammation (the ESR and CRP) are extremely helpful. The presence of profound early morning stiffness is also useful. If

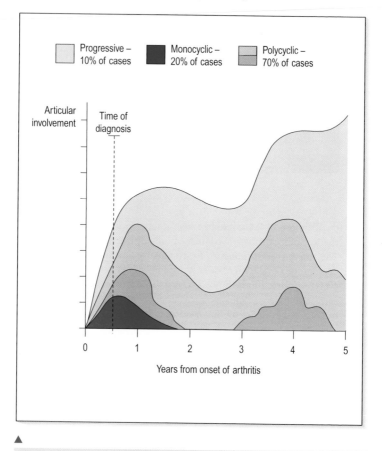

Fig. 4.2 Patterns of the clinical (articular) course of rheumatoid arthritis; articular patterns in 50 patients with rheumatoid arthritis. (From Masi et al 1983.[1])

joints are swollen then x-rays can provide a diagnosis, although if showing erosions this confirms that some damage has already occurred. If doubt still remains then either a telephone call to a rheumatologist for informal advice about referral or direct referral to a rheumatologist is important.

4.10 When should I refer a patient with suspected rheumatoid arthritis to a rheumatologist?

As a serious multisystem inflammatory disease that is associated with profound morbidity and mortality, all patients with rheumatoid arthritis should be seen and assessed by a rheumatologist. Whether long term therapy should be provided by a rheumatologist alone, shared between a rheumatologist and a primary care physician or in primary care alone will depend upon the initial assessment by a rheumatologist and, of course, local experience, expertise and facilities (*see also Ch. 10*).

It has now been clearly shown that the rheumatic disease process can best be modified and disability minimised, if treated early. It is therefore essential to refer patients with suspected RA to a rheumatologist at the earliest opportunity, where there is the maximal chance for successful intervention and disease suppression.

  PATIENT QUESTIONS

4.11 I keep asking my GP for an x-ray to see how my arthritis is doing. Why am I told this isn't needed?

Rheumatoid arthritis has usually been present for quite a long time before joint changes become apparent on an x-ray. Similarly, it can take many months or even years for a patient's x-rays to show any changes, compared to those performed previously. A much more accurate assessment of how your disease is doing is for your doctor to listen to your symptoms carefully and examine you on a regular basis.

4.12 Lots of people I know say they have arthritis – why am I much worse than them?

Most people who say they have 'arthritis' in fact have simple wear and tear in their joints. Although this wear and tear can be painful, true rheumatoid arthritis tends to be a much more significant and severe disease and, if your joints are inflamed, can cause considerable discomfort. If you are unhappy with the condition of your joints at any time then you should seek early help from the doctors and other health professionals that look after you.

4.13 My mother was crippled with rheumatoid arthritis. I have got sore joints now and I am scared that I am developing the same condition.

Rheumatoid arthritis in the past was a particularly nasty condition, because little effective treatment was available. This has changed dramatically over recent years and, today, much can be done to help patients with definite rheumatoid arthritis.

However, getting joint pains is extremely common and the vast majority of joint pains are nothing to do with rheumatoid arthritis. If you are worried that you are developing rheumatoid arthritis then it is very important that you see your doctor who will ask you more about your symptoms, examine your joints (and perhaps other parts of your body) and perform some blood tests to see if there are any of the typical features of inflammation in your blood that occur in rheumatoid arthritis. If your doctor thinks that you might be developing rheumatoid arthritis, referral to a rheumatologist who specialises in this condition can be arranged in order to check the diagnosis and, if required, start you on treatment to suppress the disease and make you feel better.

It is, however, more likely that somebody with joint pains has not got rheumatoid arthritis, even if other members of the family have it. For peace of mind, ask your doctor to check you over and if you or the doctor remain concerned, to arrange referral to a rheumatologist.

Drug treatment – symptom relief

5

5.1 Are simple analgesics helpful in rheumatoid arthritis?

Simple analgesics such as paracetamol, codeine and dextropropoxyphene (*see Appendix 3*) will help relieve pain in rheumatoid arthritis (RA) but will have no effect on the underlying cause, namely inflammation. Simple analgesics therefore are of limited use in active inflammatory rheumatoid arthritis, since they do not treat the underlying cause, or even the symptoms of inflammation. However, as the disease progresses and responds to treatment – or even becomes 'burnt out' with regard to inflammation (*see Q. 1.17*) – simple analgesics may be considerably more useful.

Single ingredient preparations are generally preferable to compound analgesics, as the compounds rarely have any analgesic advantage and certainly complicate the treatment of overdose. Dextropropoxyphene tends to be popular particularly with older patients. This is probably because of its CNS stimulatory effect as much as its analgesic properties!

Patients need to be warned when any compound analgesic they are prescribed contains paracetamol in order to avoid other paracetamol containing preparations. The hepatotoxic effects of paracetamol in overdose are well known. The constipating effects of the opiate part of some compound analgesics may be severe enough to limit their use in elderly patients.

5.2 Is there any role for opiates in the management of rheumatoid arthritis?

As a general rule, opioid analgesic use in the management of rheumatoid arthritis should be avoided. Opioids do not treat the underlying disease or prevent joint destruction. Even the thought of opioid analgesia as medication to control joint pain in a patient with RA suggests that consultation with a rheumatologist is urgently required. It is likely in such a situation that the patient's disease needs reviewing and consideration given to the use or dose alteration of a disease-modifying agent.

5.3 How do NSAIDs work?

Non-steroidal anti-inflammatory drugs (NSAIDs; *see Appendix 3*) inhibit prostaglandin, prostacyclin and thromboxane synthesis by inhibiting the enzyme cyclo-oxygenase. Prostaglandins play a particular role in pain, inflammation and fever, thromboxanes are important for making platelets sticky and prostacyclins are important for the production of the mucus barrier in the gut (*Fig. 5.1*). Traditional NSAIDs (e.g. ibuprofen, diclofenac) non-selectively inhibit the formation of these three groups of chemicals. In addition to an anti-inflammatory effect, they may also provide cardiovascular protection by reducing platelet stickiness – but cannot be

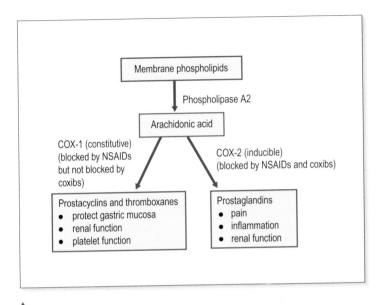

Fig. 5.1 Coxibs are able to selectively inhibit the formation of prostaglandins which mediate pain and inflammation. Conventional NSAIDs also block the formation of prostacyclins and thromboxanes important for gastroprotection and platelet function.

relied upon for this, due to relatively short half-lives, and do not replace aspirin in this role.

5.4   What role does 'COX-2' have in rheumatoid arthritis?

The enzyme cyclo-oxygenase (COX) exists in at least two forms: COX-1 and COX-2 (and also COX-3). COX-2 is involved in the production of prostaglandins, which cause inflammation and pain, and this enzyme is inducible at areas of inflammation. COX-1 is important in the production of prostacyclins (forming the protective mucous barrier in the stomach) and thromboxanes (making platelets sticky) and is constitutively expressed throughout the body.

Understanding the biology of these enzymes has led to the development of a new class of NSAIDs, the coxibs (*see Appendix 3*). These drugs selectively inhibit COX-2 and therefore suppress pain and inflammation, as do all NSAIDs, but without any excess adverse effect on damaging the protective mucosal barrier in the gut. In addition to this, the coxibs have no effect on platelet stickiness and therefore cannot replace aspirin for patients at risk of cardiovascular disease.

5.5 Are any of the available NSAIDs better for rheumatoid arthritis than any other?

On the whole, there is little difference in efficacy between available NSAIDs. The choice of these drugs for rheumatoid arthritis is based more on their duration of action and safety. In a chronic inflammatory state such as rheumatoid arthritis, drugs with a long half-life may be better for patients than drugs that need frequent dosing each day. Similarly, if patients require chronic treatment with NSAIDs then it is also important to choose ones with a better safety profile and less toxicity.

5.6 Are the 'coxibs' any better for rheumatoid arthritis than traditional NSAIDs?

Many studies[1–3] have shown that coxibs (e.g. celecoxib, etoricoxib, rofecoxib) work just as well as traditional NSAIDs in treating pain and inflammation in rheumatoid arthritis. They are, however, more expensive than traditional NSAIDs. The coxibs are, with little to choose between them, safer on the gut than traditional NSAIDs but they have a similar side effect profile with regard to other organs as do traditional NSAIDs. The National Institute for Clinical Excellence (NICE) in the UK have ruled that coxibs should be used only in patients at significant risk of gastrointestinal disease (*Box 5.1*).

5.7 What risks are associated with NSAID use?

There is much controversy surrounding the concomitant use of H_2 antagonists or proton-pump inhibitors in patients using NSAIDs. As a

---

BOX 5.1 NICE guidance on the use of COX-2 selective inhibitors for the treatment of osteoarthritis and rheumatoid arthritis

- COX-2 selective inhibitors available at time of review: rofecoxib, celecoxib, etodolac and meloxicam
- COX-2 selective inhibitors are not recommended for routine use in patients with rheumatoid arthritis or osteoarthritis
- COX-2 selective agents should be used instead of standard NSAIDs in rheumatoid arthritis or osteoarthritis when patients are at 'high risk' of developing serious gastrointestinal problems

High risk is defined as: age 65 or over; concomitant therapies which can cause gastrointestinal problems (e.g. steroids); history of gastrointestinal problems (such as ulcers); significant co-morbidity (such as cardiovascular disease, diabetes); prolonged use of maximum dose of standard NSAIDs required.

general rule, patients with a history of proven peptic ulcer disease should avoid all non-steroidals if possible. If a non-steroidal were deemed necessary in a patient with a previous history of peptic ulcer disease, NICE recommend[4] that a coxib (selective COX-2 inhibitor) should be used instead or prophylaxis against further ulceration instituted, via the concomitant prescription of a proton-pump inhibitor.

Some NSAIDs (e.g. Arthrotec) also contain misoprostol, a synthetic analogue of prostaglandin E1, as a gastroprotective agent. Misoprostol is contraindicated in women who are or who wish to become pregnant because of the risk of premature labour.

All non-steroidal anti-inflammatory drugs, including the newer coxibs, should be used with caution in patients with uncontrolled hypertension, renal failure or cardiac failure in order to avoid decompensation due to renal prostanoid blockade.

Unless absolutely necessary, co-prescription of non-steroidals with anticoagulant agents such as warfarin is best avoided. If NSAIDs are essential (as is often the case in RA, where they may provide lifelines for patients), then coxibs should be used with relative safety, raising the international normalised ratio (INR) by a fairly predictable modest 10% and, with the most recent coxibs, no effect on platelets.

Non-steroidal anti-inflammatory drugs should also be avoided in the later stages of pregnancy as they can delay the onset and increase the duration of labour. Non-steroidals may lead to in utero closure of the ductus arteriosus. All non-steroidals except aspirin can be used safely by lactating mothers.

5.8   What side effects are associated with NSAID use?

As is well known, gastrointestinal toxicity is the most worrying common side effect of NSAIDs. Inflammation, erosions and ulceration, with perforation and bleeds, can occur anywhere in the oesophagus, stomach and small bowel.

Misoprostol protects against peptic ulcers but there is a high incidence of abdominal pain and diarrhoea with its use.

The side effects of NSAID use are summarised in *Box 5.2*.

5.9   If I think a patient has rheumatoid arthritis, is it worth a trial of an NSAID prior to referral?

Any patient with sore inflamed joints would hope to receive some benefit from an NSAID. Although this type of drug will not modify the course of the disease or significantly suppress any inflammation it will certainly help with symptoms. It is therefore important to prescribe NSAIDs for patients with probable rheumatoid arthritis pending formal assessment by a rheumatologist.

BOX 5.2 Side effects of non-steroidal anti-inflammatory drugs

- Gastrointestinal tract
  — dyspepsia and gastritis
  — gastric or duodenal ulceration
  — diarrhoea
  — hepatitis
- Central nervous system
  — headache and dizziness
  — tinnitus
  — confusion
  — aseptic meningitis
- Cardiovascular system
  — oedema
  — hypertension
  — heart failure
- Respiratory system
  — asthma
  — pneumonitis
- Blood
  — neutropenia
  — thrombocytopenia
  — aplastic anaemia
  — haemolytic anaemia
- Kidney
  — precipitation of acute renal failure
  — haematuria
  — nephrotic syndrome
  — papillary necrosis
  — interstitial nephritis
- Hypersensitivity reactions

5.10 Once a patient has been referred to a rheumatologist, does the use of NSAIDs interfere with assessment of either diagnosis or treatment?

Non-steroidal anti-inflammatory drugs do not mask disease in rheumatoid arthritis and do not interfere with its diagnosis or treatment. Indeed, it is important from the patient's perspective to have a drug that will help relieve symptoms at the earliest opportunity, but not interfere with diagnosis or further treatment.

5.11 What is the role of intra-articular steroids in rheumatoid arthritis and is there a maximum number of times they can be used?

Injection of a steroid directly into an inflamed joint is an important mechanism for treating rheumatoid arthritis. Clearly, in rheumatoid arthritis, many joints can be affected at once and it is not practical to inject all of them – nor desirable by the patient! However, the occasional sore swollen inflamed joint can be settled quite quickly by aspirating fluid and injecting steroid. There are risks in injecting steroids, the most important of which are causing septic arthritis and osteoporosis, and aggravating development of osteoarthritis and skin atrophy.

There is no hard and fast rule about the number of times that joints can be injected with steroids. The most important thing is that it is done safely and appropriately. A frequent need for joint injections, however, indicates that the baseline disease-modifying anti-rheumatic therapy is inadequate and either the dosage needs increasing or the drug needs changing. Joint injections are therefore not a treatment on their own for rheumatoid arthritis, but as an adjunct, to help patients rapidly over a flare whilst the slower acting anti-rheumatic drugs are working. As a rule of thumb, however, it would seem sensible to limit the injections to an individual joint to no more than three times a year.

Intra-articular steroid injections are usually safe. However, it is helpful to provide written details to patients who have such injections with the aim of identifying potential complications at the earliest stage and minimising future problems. An example of such information is provided in *Figure 5.2.*

5.12 Which corticosteroid is best for intra-articular use?

There is again no hard and fast rule here. Long acting drugs such as methylprednisolone are, however, usually used for injection of large joints. The use of hydrocortisone is preferable when injecting superficial joints or flexor tendon sheaths as this weaker steroid preparation is associated with a lower incidence of subcutaneous and skin atrophy.

5.13 What are the risks of joint injections?

Even in the most experienced of hands and the most ideal conditions, there are risks to the patient of having their joints injected with a steroid. Indeed, merely introducing a needle into a joint without injecting anything can cause a problem such as sepsis. The risk of causing the problem increases

STEROID INJECTIONS

- You have been given a steroid injection today. This has a powerful anti-inflammatory effect on painful tendons, muscles and joints. This effect builds up over three to four days.

- The area may be more painful for a few days. You may need to take one or two tablets of paracetamol, or your usual painkiller, to help the pain.
  N.B. Follow the instructions on the container or on the leaflet in the box.

- It is important that you follow the instructions that you have been given about exercising the joint.

Are there any complications of having this injection?

There may be a small amount of discomfort. Side-effects are rare but may occur.
These include:

- If you experience any pain or discomfort it usually subsides within a few days (see above).
- Some patients experience facial flushing. Do not worry as this usually subsides within a day or two.
- Diabetic patients need to monitor their blood/urine sugars as these may rise. Diet and medication may have to be adjusted for a few days following the injection.
- Some women find that there is some irregularity of the menstrual cycle following the injection. This may be in the form of break-through bleeding or a missed period. If you are concerned, please contact your GP.
- Sometimes the injection fluid can leak back and cause some skin irritation and, on rare occasions, skin thinning.
- Occasionally, the site of the injection can become infected: this is extremely rare. Signs of developing infection include the area becoming sore and starting to throb after the first 24 hours. Sometimes it will look red and angry. If either of these problems occur, or you are concerned for any reason, then contact a doctor on the same day to check whether treatment is needed.

▲

Fig. 5.2 Example of instructions to patient following steroid injection.

with inexperience in joint injections and performing them in inappropriate settings, where aseptic technique cannot be performed.

The potential side effects of joint injections include:

- sepsis (which may occur quickly or be masked if steroids are injected)
- joint damage
- haemarthrosis (especially if patients are taking warfarin or another anticoagulant)
- osteoporosis
- atrophy of subcutaneous tissues in skin
- tendon rupture
- a crystal arthritis (rarely).

5.14 What is the role of bolus IV or IM steroids in rheumatoid arthritis?

On the whole, most rheumatologists prefer to avoid chronic steroid therapy in rheumatoid arthritis because of the unacceptable side effects. However, occasional steroid usage can be extremely helpful. A patient presenting with particularly severe disease with many joints involved or a patient flaring up with lots of other organs involved in rheumatoid arthritis may benefit from a brief hospital admission with intravenous bolus of high dose methylprednisolone. This may be helpful to rapidly suppress severe disease. However, it should not be performed lightly, because of major potential adverse effects, which include inducing a negative protein balance, reducing bone density and increasing the chance of diabetes and serious sepsis – all of which are compounded with repeated infusions or injections.

An alternative and preferred way of delivering occasional steroid is by intramuscular deposteroid injections with, for example, methylprednisolone acetate (Depo-Medrone). Since most disease modifying anti-rheumatic drugs work slowly, it is often helpful for a newly diagnosed patient just started on a disease-modifying drug to have an intramuscular injection of an average of 120 mg of Depo-Medrone. This will help suppress joint inflammation within a couple of days and last anything from between 2 weeks and 2 months. This injection should not be given before referral to a rheumatologist, as it can mask signs and symptoms and make diagnosis more difficult. Again, if not repeated too frequently and if used to help re-establish remission this can be a useful way of helping patients, but should not replace the disease-modifying anti-rheumatic drug as main therapy for rheumatoid arthritis.

5.15 Do you think steroid injection should be the preserve of secondary care?

Steroids should not be used whilst a patient is waiting to see a rheumatologist for diagnosis as steroid can mask symptoms and signs. However, this might be hard to resist if there is a particularly long waiting list for a rheumatologist. Similarly, if the patient with rheumatoid arthritis is flaring and the background anti-rheumatic medication is ineffective it is important that the rheumatologist knows this, as he or she will be in the best position to change therapy. In this case, an expedited appointment for a rheumatologist may be preferable to a deposteroid injection being given in primary care. Additionally, there are a number of side effects of deposteroid injections, ranging from fat atrophy to osteoporosis if the cumulative dose is high enough. It is not therefore a treatment modality that should be considered often in primary care without considerable experience in the management of RA.

5.16 What is the role of oral steroids in rheumatoid arthritis?

There is ongoing debate as to the role of oral steroids in rheumatoid arthritis. These drugs were used extensively in the past where they clearly helped suppress joint inflammation but ultimately at the cost of many side effects, ranging from diabetes through hypertension to osteoporosis. Some recent work has shown that low dose steroids can work quite effectively in mild rheumatoid arthritis, without causing side effects (e.g. 10 mg of prednisolone). However, with the advent of effective disease-modifying anti-rheumatic drugs that are clearly able to suppress disease and without major side effects if given carefully, the role of oral steroids in rheumatoid arthritis is extremely limited, and not recommended for primary care.

Occasionally, oral steroids may be useful in the older patient in whom a high quality of life is important but long term co-morbidity is not. Oral steroids should not be given before formal diagnosis by a rheumatologist as this can certainly mask symptoms and signs.

Finally, it is much harder to get a patient off oral steroids than if these drugs are given intramuscularly; additionally, the cumulative dose exposure may be higher if steroid is given orally.

PATIENT QUESTIONS

5.17   Is injecting my joints with steroids dangerous?

Many people worry about regular use of steroids of any type, their biggest concern being the possibility of gaining weight. We may also be familiar with stories of footballers who have been 'crippled' because they were injected with steroids during their playing careers. Unless you are allergic to the drug, having your joints injected on an infrequent basis, by someone who knows what they are doing, may well be of benefit to you and is unlikely to pose you any problems. The infrequent injection of steroid directly into your joints is not associated with the same side effects as long term use of steroid tablets. In terms of our crippled footballers, most of these problems relate to the inappropriate injection of steroid into ligaments/tendons and not into joints!

5.18   I feel better since my doctor gave me painkillers. Do I still need to see a specialist?

In short, yes. All patients with rheumatoid arthritis should be assessed by a consultant rheumatologist in order to ensure that the most appropriate treatment is being given. Looking after patients with rheumatoid arthritis is a partnership between lots of different people (doctors, nurses, therapists, etc.) and sometimes only hospital rheumatology departments are able to provide particular treatments that may be essential to help you.

5.19   Why are my joints worse in cold/damp weather?

This question has puzzled doctors for very many years. Nearly every patient with an inflammatory joint problem claims that 'bad weather' makes the affected joints worse. It is not cold and damp themselves which would appear to be the problem but possibly a fall in barometric pressure. There are certain nerve receptors in our joints which respond to pressure changes. In the UK, a falling barometric pressure is usually associated with increasing cloud and rain and this may explain why patients associate this type of weather with bad joints. In other parts of the world, a falling barometric pressure will be associated with deteriorating joints even if the sun is shining!

Drug treatment – disease modifiers/suppressants

INTRODUCTION

6.1 Does early intervention with DMARDs improve outcome?

In the past, it has been a sad reflection on rheumatology that few adequately designed studies have been performed to detect any significant objective benefit on the course of disease by treating rheumatoid arthritis. Patients were told, 'there is nothing more that can be done for you'. This has now changed. There is now a huge body of evidence accruing to show, quite clearly, that the early diagnosis and early aggressive intervention by disease-modifying anti-rheumatic drugs (DMARDs) can significantly slow or even halt disease and certainly really improve outcome.[1,2]

Outcome is better from the patients' perspective of their quality of life, by independent functional assessments of patients, and by objective measurements of joint damage from x-rays and reduction of inflammation by blood tests. However, it is also clear, in parallel, that anti-rheumatic therapy with disease-modifying drugs can now suppress disease activity extremely well but only very rarely can it 'cure' disease. Therefore, when these drugs are stopped, there is a tendency for disease to flare up again and, to this extent, rheumatoid arthritis can be compared to insulin dependent diabetes, where early diagnosis and good disease control with insulin can result in normal lives, but when insulin is stopped the disease flares up again and poor control of disease leads to complications and organ damage.

6.2 What combinations of DMARD treatment are common?

As for cancer, it is possible that treating rheumatoid arthritis by a combination of drugs works better than just giving a single drug on its own. However, most patients today are started on methotrexate and if this drug does not work, patients may have either sulfasalazine or, more recently, leflunomide added into their treatment.

Addition of hydroxychloroquine to methotrexate and sulfasalazine constitutes so-called 'triple therapy' which has been shown, in some studies, to work better than a single agent in patients with severe disease.[3]

6.3 When used in combination, do DMARDs work independently or synergistically?

The body of evidence to date[3] suggests that a combination of drugs may work better than a single drug on its own. Almost certainly, there is likely to be a degree of synergy; however more work is required to fully address this question.

SULFASALAZINE

6.4 How does sulfasalazine work?

Sulfasalazine was one of the first drugs originally designed to treat rheumatoid arthritis. It was developed from the theory that rheumatoid arthritis is caused by an infection and also that aspirin helps treat its symptoms. The drug therefore is a combination of a sulphonamide antibiotic coupled to an aspirin derivative. This drug certainly works, suppressing disease activity in rheumatoid arthritis, but probably for different reasons. The real reasons why sulfasalazine works as a disease-modifying drug in rheumatoid arthritis remain unknown.

6.5 What dosage should be given?

Sulfasalazine is usually given in a total dose of 2–3 g per day in two divided doses, and the dosage gradually built up to reduce side effects. It can take up to 3 months for this drug to produce a clinical benefit.

6.6 What are the side effects of sulfasalazine?

 Severe side effects to sulfasalazine are normally rare. The most common side effect is that of bloating or nausea with headaches or diarrhoea. In order to reduce these side effects, sulfasalazine should be started at 500 mg once a day and increased in weekly increments up to a stable dose of usually 2 g per day. In more resistant disease, 3 g a day can be given. Most patients prefer to take this drug in two divided doses.

Sulfasalazine can rarely cause liver damage or bone marrow suppression. It can also cause skin rashes and a reversible oligospermia.

6.7 What blood tests are important in monitoring and how often should these be done?

In order to maintain and ensure safety in dosage of sulfasalazine it is recommended that patients have regular blood tests for full blood count (FBC) and liver function. It is usually acceptable for liver function tests to rise slightly, but as long as enzymes do not go higher than three times the upper limit of normal it is safe to continue.

Monitoring for sulfasalazine is usually performed at 3-monthly intervals, but more frequently when becoming established on it. Current recommendations for monitoring this and the other DMARDs described below are listed in *Table 6.1*.

PENICILLAMINE

6.8 How does penicillamine work?

It is not known how penicillamine works as a disease-modifying drug in rheumatoid arthritis. There was greater usage of penicillamine in the past, because it has a definitive disease-modifying effect. However, this drug is given rarely today, because of the relatively high frequency of side effects and the availability of other drugs, which work just as well, if not better, and have fewer side effects. Penicillamine starts to reduce remission during a period of 3–6 months.

6.9 What dosage should be given?

Penicillamine is usually started at 125 mg a day and increased up to a usual maintenance dose of between 500 and 750 mg a day.

6.10 What are the side effects of penicillamine?

 Penicillamine can commonly cause loss of taste or a metallic taste together with nausea and rashes. Isolated cytopenias can be found and renal impairment with proteinuria and haematuria, which can occur in up to 30% of patients. However, this may resolve despite continuation of treatment as long as renal function tests remain normal, oedema is absent and there is no significant increase in proteinuria.

Rare side effects include aplastic anaemia, agranulocytosis, haemolytic anaemia, systemic lupus erythematosus-like syndrome, myasthenia gravis-like syndrome, pemphigus, and Goodpasture's and Stevens–Johnson syndromes.

6.11 What blood tests are important in monitoring and how often should these be done?

Urinalysis and FBC with renal function tests should be carried out every 2 weeks until on a stable dose and then monthly thereafter. Patients should be asked about the presence of a rash or mouth ulcers at each visit.

HYDROXYCHLOROQUINE

6.12 How does hydroxychloroquine work?

It is not known how hydroxychloroquine works in rheumatoid arthritis. There is evidence, though, that it is able to reduce symptoms and act as a relatively weak disease-modifying drug. Its effect takes about 3–6 months to become apparent. It is most unusual for this drug to be used on its own in the management of established rheumatoid arthritis. It is almost always used in combination with other disease-modifying drugs.

6.13 What dosage should be given?

The most usual dose is 200 mg once a day.

6.14 What are the side effects of hydroxychloroquine?

 Side effects are extremely rare with hydroxychloroquine, although some patients experience gastrointestinal disturbances.

Rare side effects include headache, visual disturbances, corneal opacities, hypopigmentation of skin or loss of hair, and ECG changes.

6.15 What blood tests are important in monitoring and how often should these be done?

There is no need to monitor blood tests for hydroxychloroquine. This may be very helpful in some patients who are not able to attend for blood monitoring of potential DMARD side effects.

Some rheumatologists and ophthalmologists advocate yearly visual screenings to detect ocular toxicity – although the true requirement and benefit of this is extremely low.

SODIUM AUROTHIOMALATE

6.16 How does sodium aurothiomalate work?

Sodium aurothiomalate, or injectable gold, has been shown to work well as a disease-modifying drug in rheumatoid arthritis. How it works is totally unknown, in common with most traditional disease-modifying drugs, although it does have effects on a variety of immune cells. Gold takes up to 3 months to have a clinical effect.

6.17 What dosage should be given?

Gold is administered intramuscularly. A test dose of 10 mg is given in the first instance. If there is no reaction to this with allergy or other side effects, then it is given as weekly injections of 50 mg intramuscularly until remission and then the interval between injections is extended to either fortnightly or monthly. In the past, gold was stopped when a certain cumulative dose was reached. Today, it is continued – but carefully monitored and with an increased interval between doses.

6.18 What are the side effects of sodium aurothiomalate?

 Gold is particularly prone to cause a variety of side effects ranging from an allergic rash, which might extend to erythroderma, through to renal involvement with proteinuria and haematuria (and ultimately renal failure). It may also cause significant bone marrow suppression.

Rare side effects include colitis, peripheral neuritis, pulmonary fibrosis, hepatotoxicity and alopecia.

6.19 What blood tests are important in monitoring and how often should these be done?

Because of the high risk of toxicity from gold this drug is used rarely in rheumatoid arthritis today. It is advised that patients on gold therapy have a FBC and urinalysis before each gold injection – although the results do not need to be available on the same day as the injection and it is acceptable to work one FBC 'in arrears'.

Monitoring should be carried out at the same frequency as the injection of gold (i.e. weekly to monthly).

AURANOFIN

6.20 How does auranofin work?

Auranofin is an oral preparation of gold. As for injectable gold it has effects on a variety of immune cells but the reason it may help in rheumatoid arthritis is not known. Auranofin has a very weak (if any) disease-modifying effect in rheumatoid arthritis, which takes from 4–6 months to come on. It is very rarely used today.

6.21 What dosage should be given?

Auranofin is administered only on expert advice, at a dose of 6 mg per day. It is administered initially in two divided doses and then, if tolerated, as a single dose. If response is inadequate after 6 months, the dose can be increased to 9 mg daily, in three divided doses; discontinue if there is no response after a further 3 months.

6.22 What are the side effects of auranofin?

 Common side effects are diarrhoea and low white cell counts, with rashes and/or mouth ulcers.

Rarely auranofin can cause the wider profile of side effects as observed for intramuscular sodium aurothiomalate.

6.23 What blood tests are important in monitoring and how often should these be done?

Full blood count should be performed every month. Patients should be asked about the presence of a rash or mouth ulcers at each visit.

CICLOSPORIN

6.24 How does ciclosporin work?

Ciclosporin was originally used in organ transplantation as an anti-T-cell drug to suppress organ rejection. It has a disease-modifying effect in rheumatoid arthritis, probably because of its ability to suppress T-cells, which are important white blood cells in orchestrating the immune response. It takes from 6 weeks to 3 months to produce a clinical benefit.

6.25 What dosage should be given?

Ciclosporin is usually given at a dose of between 2 and 5 mg per kg per day in two divided doses to treat rheumatoid arthritis.

6.26 What are the side effects of ciclosporin?

 Ciclosporin may cause a dose dependent increase in serum creatinine and hypertension which, undetected, may lead to renal damage. It also commonly causes gingival hyperplasia and hirsutism.

Rare side effects include a burning sensation in hands and feet, headache, rash, anaemia, hyperkalaemia, hypercholesterolaemia, hyperuricaemia, gout, pancreatitis, increase in weight, confusion, paraesthesia, convulsions and potentially a higher incidence of malignancies and lymphoproliferative disorders.

6.27 What blood tests are important in monitoring and how often should these be done?

Monitoring of ciclosporin involves fortnightly blood tests, which include FBC and creatinine and blood pressure measurement. A creatinine clearance should be established before commencement of ciclosporin. Increase of serum creatinine above 20% of the baseline creatinine is an indication to stop ciclosporin. Similarly, an increase in blood pressure may lead to cessation of therapy but it is acceptable, if appropriate, to treat hypertension with drugs such as nifedipine to maintain patients on ciclosporin if effective.

Blood tests should be performed fortnightly until stable for 3 months and then monthly thereafter.

AZATHIOPRINE

6.28 How does azathioprine work?

Azathioprine has an effect on a variety of immune system cells. It is of some use as a disease-modifying drug in rheumatoid arthritis, but is one of the weaker drugs in this role. It is likely that it works by suppressing T-cell function. It starts to work from 2–3 months of commencing therapy.

6.29 What dosage should be given?

Azathioprine is usually given in rheumatoid arthritis at doses of between 100 and 300 mg per day.

6.30 What are the side effects of azathioprine?

 The most common side effect of azathioprine is nausea.

Rare side effects include dose related bone marrow suppression, hair loss, increased susceptibility to infections in patients also receiving corticosteroids, nausea, pancreatitis, pneumonitis and disturbed liver function.

6.31 What blood tests are important in monitoring and how often should these be done?

It is advised that patients taking azathioprine for rheumatoid arthritis should have a FBC weekly for the first month and then monthly thereafter. Liver function tests should be performed monthly.

CYCLOPHOSPHAMIDE

6.32 How does cyclophosphamide work?

Cyclophosphamide is a cytotoxic drug, which is used in relatively low doses in rheumatoid arthritis. It has a weak role in suppressing synovitis and is not usually used as a disease-modifying drug in RA.

6.33 What dosage should be given?

In high doses, however, cyclophosphamide has an important role in treating systemic rheumatoid vasculitis, which may complicate rheumatoid arthritis. Cyclophosphamide should only be given in secondary care for RA (or indeed any other indications) and is given either continuously in low doses orally or (preferably) intermittently as IV (or oral) in very high boluses, together with methylprednisolone.

6.34 What are the side effects of cyclophosphamide?

 Cyclophosphamide can cause infertility, premature menopause, a tendency to bladder cancer and to severe sepsis.

6.35 What blood tests are important in monitoring and how often should these be done?

 Cyclophosphamide is a particularly dangerous drug to be used in any way in primary care and therefore monitoring for this drug would be performed exclusively within secondary care.

METHOTREXATE

6.36 How does methotrexate work?

Methotrexate is considered as the gold standard conventional disease-modifying anti-rheumatic drug today. It has been shown clearly to work as a disease-modifying drug by reducing symptoms and disease activity and it is also relatively safe. As with most other current anti-rheumatic drugs the reason it works is not known. It has certainly had an effect on many immune system cells (and indeed other cells) but why it is particularly good in rheumatoid arthritis is not known. It starts to work after 1–3 months of therapy.

6.37 What dosage should be given?

Methotrexate is given once a week by oral, intramuscular or subcutaneous injection. The usual starting dose is 10 mg per week and the dose can be increased, if tolerated and safe, up to approximately 30 mg per week in some patients. In the UK, to avoid some of the toxicity of methotrexate, folic acid is co-administered at a dose of 5 mg per day for 5 days a week (usually not taken on the same day the methotrexate is taken). It is essential to remember that methotrexate is administered only once a week and that severe toxicity can occur if, by mistake, it is taken daily.

6.38 What are the side effects of methotrexate?

Methotrexate can commonly cause a little nausea and it is therefore usually advised that this drug be taken in the evening, where nausea might not be an issue as patients sleep. It may also cause liver function abnormalities.

Methotrexate can rarely cause liver damage and cirrhosis. This is an extremely rare complication in rheumatoid arthritis in the dosage given, but something that can be and must be monitored for. Similarly, methotrexate can cause an acute inflammatory pneumonitis, which may be life threatening.

Methotrexate has a mild effect on suppressing the immune system, and may make some patients a little more susceptible to disease. Some patients experience a profound worsening of rheumatoid nodules when taking methotrexate.

6.39 What blood tests are important in monitoring and how often should these be done?

It is advised that patients taking methotrexate have a fortnightly FBC and liver function test analysis for the first month or after each dosage increase, and then monthly thereafter. Liver enzymes may be allowed to rise up to a maximum of three times the upper limit of normal before taking any action to reduce the dose or stop the drug. Similarly, a reduction of absolute white cell count below $4 \times 10^9/l$ would be an indication to review the patient and possibly stop the drug.

LEFLUNOMIDE

6.40 How does leflunomide work?

Leflunomide (*see also Q. 7.4*) affects the function of T-lymphocytes (and also other cells that are pyrimidine scavengers) and takes from 2 weeks to 3 months for its beneficial effects to become apparent.

6.41 What dosage should be given?

Dosages for leflunomide are currently under review.

6.42 What are the side effects of leflunomide?

 Leflunomide may cause hypertension, skin rashes, alopecia and diarrhoea. It can also cause liver function abnormality. A significant proportion of patients may develop troublesome complications, particularly diarrhoea. However, if the drug is given without a loading dose and started at 10 mg rather than 20 mg a day these side effects, if occurring, may be relatively transient. The plasma half-life of leflunomide is approximately 1 month and, as it is extremely teratogenic in animals, it is contraindicated in pregnancy or in patients with a significant chance of getting pregnant whilst taking this drug. If there is any risk of pregnancy or other major toxicity then the drug must be eliminated from the body by, for example, administration of colestyramine.

6.43 What blood tests are important in monitoring and how often should these be done?

It is recommended that monitoring of FBC, liver function tests and blood pressure be performed fortnightly for 1 month and then at monthly intervals as for methotrexate.

CONSEQUENCES OF DMARD TREATMENT

6.44 Do DMARDs cause cancer?

The common feature of most effective disease-modifying anti-rheumatic drugs (perhaps with the exception of sulfasalazine and hydroxychloroquine) is that they suppress the immune system. Since the immune system is important not only for protection against infection but also as part of the body's tumour surveillance mechanisms it is theoretically possible that chronic suppression of the immune system in the treatment of rheumatoid

Table 6.1   DMARDs used for the treatment of rheumatoid arthritis

DMARD	Time for clinical benefit to patient	Side effects	Monitoring
Auranofin	4–6 months	Diarrhoea Leucopenia	Monthly FBC and urinalysis Ask about rashes or oral ulceration at each visit
Azathioprine	2–3 months	Dose related bone marrow suppression Hypersensitivity (including malaise, nausea, deranged LFTs) Increased susceptibility to infection	FBC and LFTs weekly for 1 month at stable dose and then monthly thereafter
Ciclosporin	6 weeks–3 months	Dose-dependent increase in serum creatinine Hypertension Gastrointestinal disturbances Hypertrichosis Gingival hyperplasia Paraesthesia and tremor Increased susceptibility to infection and ?tumours	Serum creatinine and blood pressure fortnightly until stable dose for 3 months and then monthly thereafter FBC and LFTs monthly until dose is stable for 3 months and then 3 monthly; serum lipids 6 monthly
Hydroxychloroquine	3–6 months	Gastrointestinal disturbances Headache Skin reactions Retinal toxicity	Possible formal visual screening
Sodium aurothiomalate (IM)	3 months	Mouth ulcers, skin rash Vasomotor symptoms Leucopenia, thrombocytopenia Proteinuria, nephritic syndrome Cholestatic jaundice Peripheral neuropathy	FBC and urinalysis before each injection Ask patient about rashes or oral ulceration before each injection

Table 6.1 DMARDs used for the treatment of rheumatoid arthritis—cont'd

DMARD	Time for clinical benefit to patient	Side effects	Monitoring
Leflunomide	2 weeks–3 months	Alopecia Nausea, diarrhoea Skin rash Leucopenia, thrombocytopenia Deranged LFTs Hypertension	FBC and LFTs 2 weekly for the first month and then monthly thereafter
Methotrexate	4 weeks–3 months	Nausea, diarrhoea Mouth ulcers Alopecia Deranged LFTs, liver cirrhosis Leucopenia, thrombocytopenia Allergic pneumonitis Nodulosis	FBC and LFTs fortnightly for the first month and then monthly thereafter U&Es 6–12 monthly (more frequently if there is any reason to suspect deteriorating renal function)
Penicillamine	3–6 months	Nausea, loss of taste Bone marrow suppression Proteinuria, haematuria Autoimmune diseases	Fortnightly urinalysis and FBC until on a stable dose and then monthly thereafter Ask about rashes or oral ulceration at each visit
Sulfasalazine	3 months	Headache, dizziness Nausea, diarrhoea Mouth ulcers, rash Reversible oligospermia Deranged LFTs Bone marrow suppression	FBC fortnightly and LFTs monthly for the first 3 months and then 3 monthly thereafter Ask about rashes or oral ulceration at each visit

FBC, full blood count; LFTs, liver function tests; U&Es, urea and electrolytes arthritis increases the risk for tumour development. However, to date this does not seem to be the case in reality.

Rheumatoid arthritis itself appears to have a very slight association with increases in some malignancies such as lymphomas. When the effects of standard disease-modifying drugs are factored into this there does not appear to be any excess development of tumour. It is therefore appropriate to reassure patients, if they are concerned, that their chances of developing cancers are, at worst, only minimally higher when taking anti-rheumatic drugs than they would have been otherwise.

Similarly, it should also be understood that untreated RA can cause severe disability and an excess mortality. Therefore the risk of cancer (or other severe consequence) from the use of a DMARD should be weighed against clear benefit in suppressing disease. There is usually no problem in concluding that DMARD therapy is acceptable.

 PATIENT QUESTIONS

6.45 Why is my rheumatologist planning to start me on a major new drug?

You have been diagnosed as having rheumatoid arthritis. This is a condition which results from inflammation in your joints. If the inflammation in your joints is not suppressed it can cause damage and further pain. Your doctor has recommended you take a 'disease-modifying drug' which is used to try to suppress inflammation in your joints. This is different from the other types of drugs that you have taken for your arthritis such as simple painkillers or aspirin-like non-steroidal anti-inflammatory drugs. Those drugs help reduce pain and other symptoms but do not treat the underlying disease. It is of great importance that the underlying inflammation in your joints is suppressed. A variety of drugs – the disease-modifying anti-rheumatic drugs – work to suppress joint inflammation, thereby reducing your pain and minimising the chances of your joints becoming damaged.

6.46 What choices for disease-modifying drugs do I have?

There are a number of different disease-modifying anti-rheumatic drugs. All have been shown to be helpful in suppressing inflammation in joints and therefore treating rheumatoid arthritis itself. All work by different mechanisms and all have the chance of causing side effects. The type of side effect varies between drugs. Not everybody gets a side effect but sometimes certain drugs are not recommended because they may be more prone to give you a particular side effect. Your rheumatologist or rheumatology specialist nurse will explain to you the various options with the possible benefits and risk for each drug. Together with your rheumatologist you can then decide which drug may best suit you.

However, it is not always possible to predict which drug will suit a particular person and you may therefore have to change drugs if either you develop an unacceptable side effect or the drug does not work as well as you and your doctor would hope.

6.47 How much relief can I expect?

The aim of treating rheumatoid arthritis is to try to suppress fully all inflammation in your joints and get you feeling fit and well. This is sometimes relatively easy to achieve but other times it can be very difficult. You should therefore aim to have full suppression of your inflammation with no swollen or tender joints and no stiffness in your joints in the morning. If you have started on a disease-modifying drug and, after a reasonable period of time (which varies between the drugs) you feel you have not improved, then it is important you tell your doctor, who may then increase the dose of the drug until it works or, if it is not working at all, change you to a different drug which may suit you better.

6.48 What are the risks?

All drugs carry risks of side effects. Even dummy tablets made up of sugar in medical studies seem to cause side effects in some people! The most important thing with the disease-modifying anti-rheumatic drugs is that, almost always, the potential for side effects can be recognised very early if your doctor or nurse keeps a close eye on you by checking you over every now and then and performing regular blood tests. Any abnormalities in your blood tests can be picked up quickly and, if necessary, the dose of the drug can be reduced or stopped – before you will have noticed any problems yourself. Side effects are almost always reversible and go away after the drug has been reduced in dosage or stopped.

It is therefore of critical importance that, when you start a new anti-rheumatic drug, you agree to be checked over and have your blood tested at regular intervals as explained to you by your doctor or nurse. Your rheumatologist will not be able to start you on one of these drugs if you are not able to have these check-ups and blood tests. If, having started a new drug, you are not able to carry on with check-ups and blood tests your doctor may wish to stop the drug as its safety cannot be guaranteed.

6.49 What if it doesn't work?

There are a variety of disease-modifying anti-rheumatic drugs. If one drug does not work or causes side effects which are a problem, the drug can be changed for a different one. However, some anti-rheumatic drugs are much more effective than others and it is therefore important to try to give the drugs sufficient time to see if they are working before requesting a change and also if you do experience some side effects, to make sure that they are not just temporary problems that will go away after a short while.

If for whatever reason a drug is not suitable for you, then your doctor should be able to find an alternative. However, sometimes patients with particular medical conditions cannot be safely given some anti-rheumatic drugs and their options might be much more limited.

Similarly, if you have not responded to two, three or four of the best standard anti-rheumatic drugs your rheumatologist may recommend that you try one of the new 'biologic' anti-rheumatic drugs which have been shown to work in situations where ordinary drugs have not been successful.

Drug treatment – newer agents

7

7.1 Can antibiotics be useful in rheumatoid arthritis?

Minocycline, a relatively broad spectrum antibiotic, has been shown in a variety of clinical studies to be effective in reducing inflammation in rheumatoid arthritis. In clinical practice, however, it has a beneficial effect in only a relatively modest proportion of patients.

7.2 How does minocycline work?

It is not known whether minocycline helps rheumatoid arthritis because it is an antibiotic or because of other idiosyncratic properties of this drug. Certainly, minocycline is able to inhibit a group of chemicals called matrix metalloproteinases, which are involved in joint destruction in inflammatory arthritis. Minocycline may be used in patients with rheumatoid disease who are not able to take other disease-modifying anti-rheumatic drugs (*see Ch. 6*), perhaps because of the risk of infection or concomitant liver disease.

7.3 Are there any cautions in the use of minocycline?

Minocycline has been shown to trigger a lupus-like illness in some people. It should therefore not be given to patients with rheumatoid arthritis who are significantly positive for anti-nuclear antibodies. In addition, patients with rheumatoid arthritis taking minocycline should be checked up clinically at regular intervals of a month or so, with questions asked about symptoms of autoimmune disease and blood taken for anti-nuclear antibody and double-stranded DNA testing at regular intervals.

7.4 What is leflunomide?

Leflunomide (*see Q. 6.40*) is one of the newest orally active disease-modifying anti-rheumatic drugs (DMARDs) that has been designed to treat rheumatoid arthritis. It has now been available for some years.

7.5 How successful has leflunomide usage been to date?

Large scale, well-controlled clinical trials[1] have clearly shown that leflunomide is very capable of suppressing symptoms, underlying disease and disease progression in rheumatoid arthritis. Its effectiveness would appear to be comparable to that of methotrexate.

7.6 Is leflunomide expensive?

Leflunomide is more expensive than methotrexate (one of the cheapest DMARDs), being comparable to the cost of ciclosporin. It is, however, considerably less expensive than the new biologic anti-rheumatic drugs.

7.7 What is TNF-alpha?

Tumour necrosis factor alpha (TNF-alpha) is an inflammation chemical (cytokine) which seems to be important in inducing inflammation. This is a normal chemical, which is important in host defence and in tumour surveillance.

7.8 Why is TNF-alpha important in rheumatoid arthritis?

Over recent years, considerable research has shown that TNF-alpha levels are raised in affected joints in patients with rheumatoid arthritis and in particularly painful joints. Laboratory work has suggested that not only does TNF-alpha cause inflammation itself in rheumatoid arthritis, but it also stimulates the production of other inflammatory chemicals.[2] Animal models of arthritis have shown that inhibiting TNF-alpha causes improvement in disease.

TNF-alpha is also made in excess in many cancers and is responsible, at least in part, for the cachexia and fatigue experienced in cancers – comparable to the cachexia and fatigue that occur in rheumatoid arthritis.

7.9 What are the new biologics in rheumatoid arthritis?

New drugs have recently been introduced as treatments for rheumatoid arthritis. These are drugs that neutralise the inflammation chemicals (cytokines) TNF-alpha or interleukin 1 (IL-1) beta. Three drugs are currently available to neutralise TNF-alpha: etanercept, infliximab and adalimumab. Another drug, anakinra, neutralises IL-1 beta.

- *Etanercept*: Etanercerpt is a chimeric molecule, which is fully human. It comprises one of the natural receptors for TNF-alpha coupled to the constant fragment of a human antibody. This drug binds to free TNF-alpha in the body and neutralises it.
- *Infliximab and adalimumab*: These drugs are antibodies. In infliximab the variable part of the antibody has been designed to bind to TNF-alpha and is derived from a mouse antibody. The constant part of the antibody is human. In adalimumab, the whole antibody, both the variable and the constant part, are fully human. Infliximab and adalimumab neutralise free TNF-alpha but, in contrast to etanercept, also may kill cells that have TNF-alpha on their cell surface. Whether this difference is clinically significant remains a matter of speculation.
- *Anakinra*: Anakinra is a natural human receptor antagonist to the inflammation chemical IL-1 beta. Anakinra binds to free IL-1 beta in the body and neutralises it.

7.10 How are biologics given in rheumatoid arthritis?

Etanercept is given as subcutaneous injections twice a week. Etanercept can be used on its own, or together with another disease-modifying agent such as methotrexate.

Adalimumab, the most recently licensed biologic TNF-alpha therapy in the UK, is also given by subcutaneous injection. It is administered once a fortnight but may also be given once a week. Adalimumab may be given with or without methotrexate. Infliximab is given as an intravenous infusion every 2 months (*see Fig. 7.1*), starting off at 2-weekly intervals. Infliximab must be given together with methotrexate.

Anakinra is given by daily subcutaneous injection.

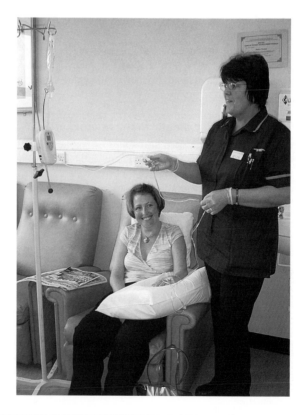

▲

Fig. 7.1 Infusion of infliximab, a monoclonal anti-TNF-alpha drug, in a patient with rheumatoid arthritis.

7.11   Do biologic drugs work in rheumatoid arthritis?

The new biologic agents, especially the anti-TNF-alpha agents, have been a major step forward in the treatment of rheumatoid arthritis. They are amongst the most potent drugs currently available that are able to suppress disease. Some studies have shown that these drugs can totally prevent further disease progression as measured by x-rays. The key clinical trial studies of these drugs have involved patients in whom all other treatments have failed. In these trials the majority have responded to these biologic agents. Clinical experience is bearing out the extremely high effectiveness of these drugs.

7.12   Are the biologic drugs prescribable in primary care?

Biologic anti-rheumatic drugs at present are only prescribable in secondary care because of the various forms of delivery for them, the potential side effects (*Box 7.1*), requirement for specialised back-up and support, and their cost. It is not anticipated that they will be suitable for delivery in primary care in the future.

7.13   What are the risks of biologic drugs?

Because TNF-alpha is important physiologically in the defence against infection and the prevention of the development of neoplasms, there are significant risks (either practical or theoretical) of anti-TNF-alpha drugs causing an increased susceptibility to infection and a higher incidence of tumours.

There is certainly an increased incidence of infection in patients taking anti-TNF-alpha therapy. Infliximab in particular has been shown to be associated with increased tuberculosis (mainly from reactivation of old infection). In addition, patients with bronchiectasis or other chronic

---

BOX 7.1   Side effects of anti-TNF-alpha therapy

■ Practical
   — increased general susceptibility to infection
   — signs of infection masked
   — rapid onset of severe infection
   — reactivation of tuberculosis (infliximab)
   — hypersensitivity reaction during infusion (infliximab)
   — development of neutralising antibody (infliximab)
   — temporary local injection site reaction (etanercept and adalimumab)
■ Theoretical
   — increased risk of tumour development (especially lymphoma)

infections should be cautioned to not have biologic therapy, as profound systemic or localised infections may occur when taking these drugs – but without the usual symptoms and signs associated. This can sometimes make diagnosis difficult. Etanercept is not associated with increased tuberculosis but, together with the other anti-TNF-alpha drugs, can be associated with severe infections, sometimes with fewer clinical signs.

On the other hand, there has been a good experience of many patients taking biologic therapy without any observed increase in the frequency of tumours over and above what would be expected normally. However, since these drugs have not been available for more than a few years, one can conclude that the risk of tumour development in patients taking anti-TNF-alpha therapy is no higher than if they were not taking such therapy – but only within our current experience of some 5 years or so. The risks of developing tumours on chronic treatment for decades remain unknown.

7.14 What monitoring is required?

There is no set blood test monitoring for biologic agents as occurs for traditional disease-modifying drugs. However, as these drugs are known to increase the risk of significant infection (particularly tuberculosis with infliximab) and because of the theoretical risk of them increasing susceptibility to tumours (which has not been observed practically to date), it is important that patients taking these drugs have been provided with good quality, easy to understand information about signs and symptoms (particularly those of infection) to look out for and to have a close link with emergency access to specialist rheumatology units.

7.15 Have the biologic drugs been NICE approved?

Etanercept and infliximab have been scrutinised by the National Institute for Clinical Excellence (NICE). This UK body has ruled that they are cost effective drugs for use in patients with rheumatoid arthritis.[3] NICE have stipulated that these drugs are given by specialist rheumatology units and that the British Society of Rheumatology (BSR) guidelines for defining entry and exit criteria are followed.

The BSR entry and exit criteria (*Box 7.2*) are based on an objective disease scoring method, the DAS 28 score (*see Q. 3.18*), which incorporates clinical and laboratory features of inflammation in ascribing a numerical score correlating with disease activity. Only patients with a DAS 28 score of greater than 5.1 are recommended for such therapy and therapy should be discontinued at 3 months if there has not been a significant improvement. Patients must also have previously tried and failed (in a good dose) at least two 'standard' disease-modifying drugs.

BOX 7.2 British Society for Rheumatology guidelines for anti-TNF-alpha therapy

■ Active disease
 — DAS > 5.1
■ Pretreatment
 — failure of at least two DMARDs after adequate trial
■ Exclusion
 — pregnancy or breast-feeding
 — active infection
 — high risk of infection (various identified)
 — malignancy or premalignancy
■ Withdrawal
 — adverse events
 — lack of effect, DAS not improved by > 1.2 at > 3 months

Finally, the NICE guidelines stipulate that all patients given such biologic treatment have their details included on a British Society of Rheumatology national register, which is administered by the Arthritis Research Campaign Epidemiology Unit in Manchester.

7.16 Are there any new drugs under research?

Although the biologic anti-TNF-alpha and IL-1 beta drugs have been a major advance, they are not wonder drugs. They are expensive, and they have already been found to have a number of practical side effects with more theoretical side effects (*see Box 7.1*), although the latter have not yet emerged. There is therefore a very active research programme both in academic medical centres and in the pharmaceutical industry to identify new drugs which might eventually offer better therapies in the future.

A whole range of new drugs is under development; some of them target T-cells, others target B-cells and yet others target other cytokines including IL-12 and IL-18. One example of an anti-B-cell drug which shows some promise in rheumatoid arthritis is retuximab. This is a monoclonal anti-B-cell antibody which is given together with other cytotoxic drugs and steroids and which, in early studies, has shown to be of benefit in some patients with rheumatoid arthritis.

There is perhaps more interest in developing new drug therapies for rheumatoid arthritis now than ever before in the past and it is an exciting time of hope for patients with rheumatoid arthritis and the medical teams looking after them.

PATIENT QUESTIONS

7.17 What are biologic anti-TNF-alpha drugs?

Rheumatoid arthritis is caused by inflammation in joints. Recent scientific work has shown that a particular chemical – tumour necrosis factor alpha (TNF-alpha) – is able to cause inflammation and is present in the joints (and blood) of patients with rheumatoid arthritis in high amounts. This important finding has prompted the development of a range of drugs that have been specifically made to neutralise this chemical. These are known as biologic anti-TNF-alpha drugs.

7.18 Do the biologic drugs work in rheumatoid arthritis?

Extensive studies have shown that anti-TNF-alpha drugs (of which the three currently available are etanercept, infliximab and adalimumab) are all able to suppress disease in rheumatoid arthritis. What is even more exciting is that most of the medical studies used to evaluate these drugs have focused on patients who have not responded to any other standard drug. In these patients, who otherwise would have no other option for treatment, more than two-thirds have responded well to the anti-TNF-alpha drugs. They therefore work extremely well in rheumatoid arthritis but are not suitable for everybody.

The National Institute for Clinical Excellence, a major body in the United Kingdom which is responsible for considering medical and surgical therapies, have formally evaluated these drugs and ruled that they are effective treatments for patients with rheumatoid arthritis who have not responded to ordinary anti-rheumatic drugs.

7.19 What are the risks of these drugs?

Biologic anti-TNF-alpha drugs work by neutralising the inflammation chemical TNF-alpha in the body. This chemical is not present just to cause rheumatoid arthritis – it is rather there to help the body fight off infections and, possibly, also to help fight off various cancers. Anti-TNF-alpha drugs may weaken the immune system a little and therefore make people more susceptible to infections. Your doctor will therefore not recommend this type of treatment if you suffer from chronic infections such as bronchiectasis. Similarly, patients with rheumatoid arthritis taking this drug may develop, rarely, severe infections. If this is the case, you must go urgently to your doctor for treatment of this infection.

Some types of anti-TNF-alpha therapy (notably infliximab) have been associated with a higher incidence of tuberculosis. If you are recommended to take this treatment you will be checked over carefully for any evidence of having this disease before starting this treatment. You may need a course of antibiotics to make sure that this infection does not turn out to be a problem.

Theoretically, anti-TNF-alpha therapies may be associated with an increased development of cancers. However, there is now good experience of these drugs being used in many thousands (if not tens of thousands) of patients over some 5 years or so. During this time there have been no extra cancers seen over and above what would be expected. We can therefore conclude that for at least 5 years or so, treatment with anti-TNF-alpha drugs do not cause cancers. However, since the drugs have only been available for a few years, it is not possible to say if they may cause problems in the longer term.

As with everything else regarding drug treatment it is always important to balance the need to have a drug (such as bad rheumatoid arthritis, which has not responded to any other drug) with the risk of side effects (which are theoretically possible for any drug). In the biologic anti-TNF-alpha therapies side effects are minimised if patients are carefully selected and looked after closely.

Non-drug treatment in rheumatoid arthritis

8

8.1 Can exercise help in rheumatoid arthritis?

Exercise is very important in rheumatoid arthritis (RA). A particular problem in RA is muscle weakness and wasting. This occurs as a combination of lack of use of joints and the excess secretion of cachetic cytokines, such as tumour necrosis factor alpha (TNF-alpha), which occurs in this disease. Maintaining a good muscle bulk is important for protecting joints, for patients' general health and for minimising loss of function. However, the timing and type of exercise will differ with the stage of disease, the type of patient and whether or not there is an active flare. Physiotherapists provide essential help in teaching exercise programmes to patients and advising them when to exercise and when to rest (*see Q. 8.11*).

8.2 Is there a recommended diet for rheumatoid arthritis?

The idea that manipulation of diet may alter symptoms in rheumatoid arthritis has been around for decades. There is, however, very little objective evidence to suggest that any particular diet is good or bad for rheumatoid arthritis. Most studies in this area have been poorly designed and have produced inadequate and uncontrolled data.

There is certainly no evidence that dietary manipulation changes the natural course of the disease but in some recent studies patients have claimed at least partial symptom relief as the result of dietary manipulation. In general terms, any condition where there tends to be an overall catabolic state would warrant a healthy diet where a sensible balance of protein, carbohydrate, fat and vitamins is important.

Dietary manipulation for rheumatoid arthritis can essentially be divided into two types: supplementation, in which substances are added to the diet, and elimination, in which foods are removed from the diet.

8.3 Which dietary supplements have been postulated to help people with rheumatoid arthritis?

There are four main supplements that warrant discussion:

- Selenium supplements
- Extracts from New Zealand green lipped mussel
- Evening primrose oil
- Fish oils.

Some patients also claim symptom relief following the use of various vitamins, herbs, royal jelly, ginseng, garlic and honey but, as there is no evidence whatsoever regarding the beneficial effects of these agents, the authors do not regard them as warranting further discussion.

8.4   How may selenium be important?

Selenium is a trace mineral that is needed by humans only in tiny amounts. Selenium has effects on the immune system and is essential for the action of glutathione peroxidase, a powerful anti-oxidant that helps to limit the harmful effects of inflammation.

There has been much study of late regarding the role of free radicals in rheumatoid arthritis and it is through its promotion of glutathione peroxidase production that selenium is thought to have its benefits. However, trials regarding selenium have thus far not shown any benefit!

8.5   What is the evidence for taking extract of New Zealand green lipped mussel?

The extract from this shellfish has been shown to have some anti-inflammatory activity. Clinical trials to date have, however, been conflicting with regard to its effectiveness and it is not recommended for use in rheumatoid arthritis.

8.6   How may evening primrose oil be effective?

Evening primrose oil is rich in gamma linolenic acid (GLA), which is a precursor of prostaglandin E1 (PGE1) – a known anti-inflammatory agent. Current trial evidence is again conflicting and further studies will need to show a definitive benefit of evening primrose oil before the authors would recommend its usage.

8.7   Are fish oils useful?

There are now over 10 randomised controlled trials showing modest but consistent benefit of fish oils in rheumatoid disease against a background of the usual pharmacotherapy.[1] Ingestion of fish oils containing ecosapentanoic acid (EPA) and docosahexaenoic acid (DHA) decreases the production of prostaglandins, leukotrienes and thromboxanes from arachidonic acid.

Long term toxicity studies are, however, still needed as the doses of these oils postulated to cause symptom improvement are in excess of those available 'over the counter'.

Fish oil taken as cod liver oil is probably not advisable in rheumatoid arthritis – omega 3 fish oils are much more likely to be helpful as they contain more EPA. It should be remembered, however, that fish oils can make certain arthritic and non-arthritic conditions worse and should be avoided in these cases (*Box 8.1*).

> **BOX 8.1 Patients who should avoid high doses of omega 3 fish oil**
>
> ■ Patients with Raynaud's syndrome
> ■ Patients with multiple sclerosis
> ■ Patients with systemic lupus erythematosus
> ■ Patients with clotting disorders
> ■ Patients taking anti-coagulant drugs
> ■ Patients with haemophilia
> ■ Patients with epilepsy
> ■ Patients with non-insulin dependent diabetes
> ■ Patients with asthma, if sensitive to aspirin

8.8 What is the evidence for dietary elimination therapy?

Foods that have been postulated to worsen synovitis include dairy products, cereals and eggs – with little consistency and no real solid clinical trial evidence.

If these foodstuffs are eliminated from the diet and symptoms consequently improve, then they must be repeatedly reintroduced in order to discover which, if any, of them reproduce symptoms. However, such elimination programmes lack credibility in a research context unless they are confirmed by a double-blind challenge.

Proper studies regarding dietary elimination take several weeks and need to be performed in a controlled setting. In the authors' experience, this usually proves not to be the case and dietary manipulation is not recommended. It should also be remembered that extreme dietary exclusions may induce deficiency disorders!

8.9 Have any complementary medical therapies been found helpful in rheumatoid arthritis?

Many patients with rheumatoid arthritis seek help from aromatherapists, homeopaths, reflexologists and herbalists. There is no scientific evidence to support the benefit of these treatments but providing they do no harm then the authors have no objection to their patients trying these therapies if they so desire. However, in the context of a severe illness such as rheumatoid arthritis, they should be used as 'complementary' and not 'alternative' therapies.

Acupuncture is now so widely used within conventional medicine that it hardly merits the term 'complementary'. It has been shown to inhibit inflammatory chemicals. Although useful to some patients, it is generally less useful in inflammatory than in degenerative rheumatic diseases.

8.10   What about alternative therapy for rheumatoid arthritis?

Many patients report variable degrees of benefit from a whole variety of alternative therapies. There are, as yet, no studies that have shown that any form of 'alternative' therapy is able to suppress disease in rheumatoid arthritis and alter outcomes. In this respect, it is totally inadvisable for patients to have an alternative therapy at the expense of standard medical therapy.

A better way of considering things would be to use other therapeutic modalities as 'complementary' rather than 'alternative' therapies. Therefore, a whole variety of methodologies ranging from aromatherapy through acupuncture to other such treatments may be found to be very helpful in a number of patients. However, it is important to bear in mind that so-called 'standard medical therapy' has been clearly shown to beneficially affect disease outcome, whereas none of the 'alternative' or 'complementary' therapies has been shown to do so.

8.11   What is the role of physiotherapy in rheumatoid arthritis?

Physiotherapy is an essential component of care for rheumatoid arthritis. All patients with newly diagnosed rheumatoid arthritis should be referred to a physiotherapist who would:

- assess them
- teach them about joint protection
- devise a simple exercise programme to maintain appropriate muscle bulk
- explain when it is better to rest and when it is better to exercise.

Patients with established disease may often need to see a physiotherapist every now and then for additional support.

As well as manipulative therapy and devising an exercise programme for the patient, a physiotherapist may decide to employ an electrotherapeutic modality to help with the patient's pain such as ultrasound or pulsed short wave diathermy. Wax and oil baths may be used for the hands and feet whilst ice gel packs may be more appropriate for large joints.

Many patients with rheumatoid arthritis, particularly those with disease affecting large joints, benefit from hydrotherapy. Once a supervised programme of hydrotherapy exercise has been initiated, patients should be encouraged to continue their programme at a local swimming baths.

8.12   What is the role of occupational therapy in rheumatoid arthritis?

Occupational therapists, as for physiotherapists, are also crucial in the delivery of care in patients with rheumatoid arthritis. All newly diagnosed patients with rheumatoid arthritis should be introduced to occupational therapists. Occupational therapists have a particular role in relation to hand function. In some situations where joints remain particularly sore and swollen, custom made splints can be manufactured to allow patients to rest and to help ease sore joints.

In patients with more advanced disease, occupational therapists are crucial in assessing patients' overall function and in helping to provide aids to maintain their activities of daily living and, when required, their ability to continue to work. Such aids can range from sticks, splints and gadgets to help hold or grip pans etc. (*Fig. 8.1*) to, if required, stair lifts and wheelchairs.

8.13 What is the role of the appliance officer/podiatrist?

Patients with rheumatoid arthritis are especially prone to get problems in their feet, from either metatarsophalangeal (MTP) joint involvement or other forefoot and midfoot problems. Having appropriate footwear is crucial for these patients, as is the case for patients with diabetes. Referral of patients with rheumatoid arthritis to a podiatrist where practical, or appliance officer where there is no access to a podiatrist, is mandatory to

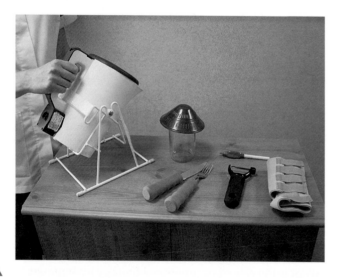

▲

Fig. 8.1 Examples of gadgets used to help maintain activities of daily living in patients with rheumatoid arthritis. These include a tip for pouring water from a kettle, a grip enhancer for opening jars, a pen grip, knife and fork grips, a potato peeler and wrist splints.

prevent worsening deformity of the feet and also to preserve mobility in patients that have severe pain when walking. Interventions can range from simple footpads to relieve pressure from MTP joints through, in some circumstances, to surgery on forefeet.

8.14　What place is there for surgery in rheumatoid arthritis?

In the past, surgeons tended to bail out rheumatologists by replacing failing joints that had been damaged by profound chronic inflammation. There is a whole range of orthopaedic interventions for rheumatoid arthritis, which is beyond the scope of this book. These range from joint replacements, through to fusions and tendon repairs to forefoot surgery. However, the onset of more aggressive and early intervention in rheumatoid arthritis is starting to have an impact on the long term course of the disease – at worst by slowing down the rate of progression and at best by putting patients into remission. Therefore, in the future, the role of orthopaedic surgery in rheumatoid arthritis may well diminish. However, it remains essential for close interactions between rheumatologists and orthopaedic surgeons to continue in order to ensure timely and correct considerations for surgery in patients with RA.

Many rheumatologists and orthopaedic surgeons run combined clinics for treating rheumatoid diseases. Such clinics are valuable for training purposes and encourage communication between the specialties, which in turn produces significant benefits in patient care.

PQ　PATIENT QUESTIONS

8.15　Will I damage my joints more if I exercise?

On the whole, exercise and moving your joints is extremely important. Joints were made to move and muscles were made to work. If these things don't happen then joints can suffer more damage or 'seize up'. However, if you have particularly acutely sore and painful joints it may not be practical to exercise much. In these situations just gentle movement of your joints will help.

It is very important that once you are diagnosed to have rheumatoid arthritis you are put in contact with a physiotherapist and an occupational therapist. The occupational therapist is very important to help you, particularly with your hands, by explaining about how to gently exercise your hands and make sure you can do the things that you wish to do. Similarly, the physiotherapist will explain to you about looking after your other joints, provide you with an exercise programme, and explain when it is important to exercise and when it is more important to rest.

8.16 Will changing my diet help my arthritis?

A lot of people claim that diets help arthritis. Many medical studies have been performed to try to investigate this but none has shown any relationship between diet and arthritis. However, as with other things in life, it is important to have a healthy diet in rheumatoid arthritis.

Being overweight can put additional stress on your joints and increase the risk of other diseases such as diabetes and heart disease. Therefore, if you are overweight it would be helpful to lose weight and, either way, to make sure that your diet contains appropriate amounts of carbohydrates, protein, roughage and not too much fat. A healthy diet with the right balance of foods including fruit should provide the right amount of vitamins.

Unless you are advised to by your doctor, there is no evidence at present to suggest you should take particular vitamins or supplements to help your arthritis.

8.17 What about glucosamine?

Glucosamine is a compound that can be taken by mouth and is claimed to help build up cartilage in joints. In osteoarthritis there is an ongoing debate as to whether this can help. In rheumatoid arthritis there is no scientific evidence at present to suggest that it helps in any way.

However, glucosamine is unlikely to cause any significant side effects if taken in moderation and, as such, whilst rheumatologists do not recommend its usage in rheumatoid arthritis they would be unlikely to mind if a patient chooses to take it.

8.18 Will I end up in a wheelchair?

Although your rheumatoid arthritis cannot be cured it can be suppressed – often fully. Relentless progression of disease is now very much the exception rather than the rule. Having a positive attitude to your disease is very important and helping yourself with regard to exercising etc. is also important. Your general practitioner, rheumatologist, nurses and therapists will do all they can to ensure you receive the best possible care. You should expect to lead a normal working and social life and have a normal life expectancy.

Social and other issues in rheumatoid arthritis

9.1 Does rheumatoid arthritis affect intercourse?

Rheumatoid arthritis can have important consequences on the personal lives of patients. Erectile dysfunction is considerably more common in men with rheumatoid arthritis than in men of comparable ages. Some of this may be due to associated depression in rheumatoid arthritis (*see Q. 9.6*) but other factors such as nerve damage and cardiovascular disease, which are higher in rheumatoid arthritis, may also contribute to this problem. Patients often do not mention this and may have significant problems that are not detected and therefore are not able to be treated.

Similarly, sore joints may obviously affect the 'mechanics' of intercourse in both males and females with rheumatoid arthritis. Again, any problems surrounding this should be enquired about and can often be helped by a combination of improving inflammatory disease control and advice about positions that might be more comfortable if joints are particularly sore. Overall libido can also be reduced as a consequence of chronic inflammatory diseases in both sexes.

9.2 Does rheumatoid arthritis affect fertility?

There are no good studies that have addressed this question adequately. Certainly, for reasons outlined above, the capacity to conceive might be reduced in patients with rheumatoid arthritis. In addition, the drugs used to treat rheumatoid arthritis may affect fertility such as the temporary oligospermia with sulfasalazine (*see Q. 6.6*).

9.3 Should pregnancies be planned in patients with rheumatoid arthritis?

It is very important that pregnancy is planned in rheumatoid arthritis. Although, on the whole, active rheumatoid arthritis is prone to remit to various degrees during pregnancy, this is not always the case.

Perhaps the most important thing to plan around pregnancy is the medication. It is critical that patients do not take a drug such as leflunomide (*see Qs 6.40 and 7.4*) with a particularly long half-life and teratogenic effects if they are planning a family. On the whole, the chance of conceiving is probably related to the degree of remission. If there is a desire to avoid potentially toxic drugs (of course the case), then temporary treatment with steroid may be the safest to avoid problems in the foetus. Non-steroidal anti-inflammatory drugs, on the whole, are relatively safe in pregnancy especially in the earlier stages and there is not so much pressure to withdraw these drugs if they are needed.

Flares of disease during pregnancy can be managed by local joint injection or, if required, by oral or parenteral steroid. The risks to the foetus from such interventions are low.

9.4   What happens on delivery of the baby?

If rheumatoid arthritis is prone to remit during pregnancy, it is also likely to flare up after delivery. This is not always the case but it is something that should be anticipated. It is recommended that there is easy access to a rheumatology service in the days or weeks immediately after delivery, as this is a time when it is particularly important to be able to care for and bond with the baby and flares of arthritis can be a serious destruction to this.

9.5   What about breast-feeding with rheumatoid arthritis?

Rheumatoid arthritis in itself is not a contraindication to breast-feeding. Many drugs that are given to treat rheumatoid arthritis can be given quite safely while breast-feeding but, as a rule of thumb, it is probably better to not take drugs apart from non-steroidal anti-inflammatory drugs in low dose.

9.6   How does the diagnosis of rheumatoid arthritis affect patients emotionally?

Having a severe systemic disease can cause many emotional and psychological problems. Patients with rheumatoid arthritis are more prone to be depressed and, as such, questions about depression should be asked and anti-depressant therapy instituted when required. Being diagnosed to have rheumatoid arthritis can be very confusing and depressing for many patients. They may be particularly scared as to whether they will end up 'crippled' and in pain. Treatment with bolus steroid by a rheumatologist on diagnosis often causes rapid and profound resolution of symptoms. This can result in patients feeling extremely optimistic about the disease – but this crashes when the disease flares up again as the steroids wear off and the disease-modifying anti-rheumatic drugs are starting to work.

It is very important that patients are provided with as much information as they can realistically cope with about the disease. Certainly a better understanding of the disease can be linked to an improved emotional state. The nature of the relapses and remissions (even with disease-modifying therapy) can be very disturbing to patients and every effort should be made to support the patient with rheumatoid arthritis while becoming established on their drugs. Similarly, flares of disease should be managed quickly and appropriately.

9.7   What does rheumatoid arthritis do to life expectancy in general?

Recent studies have shown that the development of rheumatoid arthritis can affect life expectancy to a degree comparable with that for triple vessel coronary artery disease or non-Hodgkin's lymphoma.[1] It is hoped that aggressive early therapy can minimise this effect – but it is important to bear this in mind when dealing with patients and their relatives. It also helps focus time, effort and resources in inducing as good a remission as possible and maintaining it.

9.8 What about work?

It is very important for patients with rheumatoid arthritis that they can stay at work. In some situations this might be very difficult, such as somebody who has a job that requires heavy labouring. However, it is important to temper an aggressive induction of disease remission with a realistic attitude and advice about the possibilities of maintaining gainful employment within a current job or looking to retrain to other positions.

Making major decisions about work should not be taken on immediate diagnosis of rheumatoid arthritis. It is much more important to give the patient some time to see how the disease is going to respond to treatment. Some rash decisions at diagnosis might lead to regrets if jobs are forfeited for mild disease that can be put fully into remission. The real response to treatment is what affects the capacity to work and, whilst this might become apparent in a few weeks it is more likely to take some months.

Input from occupational therapists and physiotherapists, together with counselling from rheumatology specialist nurses, is important in helping patients consider their work. For many forms of work there is not only a legal framework available to try to help people maintain their jobs but also a desire on the part of employers to help out. Close liaison with occupational health staff at the patient's place of work is important.

PATIENT QUESTIONS

9.9 Will rheumatoid arthritis affect my chances of having children?

Untreated rheumatoid arthritis can certainly affect the ability to have children. First of all, intercourse can be difficult for purely mechanical reasons if joints are very sore. In addition, if you are feeling very run down with active inflammation you may feel too tired. The profound inflammation in rheumatoid arthritis can upset a woman's menstrual cycle and, in that respect, result in a degree of infertility. In men with rheumatoid arthritis, the ability to have an erection can be impaired.

With good treatment of rheumatoid arthritis, however, most of the problems above can be removed. By suppressing the inflammation in this disease the joints will be considerably less sore, the tiredness will be not as bad and the menstrual cycle may return to normal with improved chances of conceiving.

The drug treatment of rheumatoid arthritis is very important in conception and pregnancy. Some drugs are dangerous to take while pregnant as they may cause serious problems in the baby. Other drugs (such as sulfasalazine) can temporarily reduce the sperm count, but this will go back to normal when the drug is stopped or changed and there is no effect on potency.

It is therefore very important that if you have rheumatoid arthritis and you wish to be sexually active you discuss issues around this with your doctor or nurse. While you are taking some drugs it is important that you have foolproof contraception and if you wish to get pregnant then it should be planned, so that there are no risks to you or to your baby from the disease or from the drug treatment of the disease.

9.10   What about during pregnancy and after I have a baby?

As a rule of thumb, rheumatoid arthritis is prone to improve during pregnancy. Many women with rheumatoid arthritis who become pregnant find they do not need any medication during their pregnancy. However, sometimes the disease can flare up or persistent problems occur. In these situations, it is important that you are looked after jointly by your rheumatologist and your obstetrician.

Many drugs in rheumatoid arthritis can be safely used in pregnancy but this is only recommended with appropriate specialist care.

Women who have rheumatoid arthritis may sometimes find their disease flares up on the delivery of the baby. It is therefore useful to plan an appointment with your rheumatologist for a month or so after you have delivered the baby and have a mechanism to contact the rheumatology team urgently if you have a nasty flare. Such flares can usually be suppressed very quickly and need not interfere with you looking after your new baby.

9.11   What about breast-feeding?

Breast-feeding with rheumatoid arthritis is often not a problem. However, this is an issue that you must discuss with your rheumatologist and general practitioner whilst you are pregnant. If you are feeling well and do not need any medication there should be no problems. If, however, your joints flare up you may need a variety of different medications to suppress your rheumatoid arthritis – some of which are not advisable if you are breast-feeding.

Coordinating care for the rheumatoid patient – who should do what?

10

10.1 What do rheumatology specialist nurses do?

Rheumatology specialist nurses play a very important role in the management of rheumatoid arthritis. Whilst doctors may be good at making a diagnosis, and instituting and changing treatment, nurses are perhaps the best at delivering treatment, educating patients and monitoring for toxicity.

The role of the rheumatology specialist nurse has expanded dramatically over recent years. In our centre, rheumatology nurses are instrumental in:

- educating patients about arthritis (which has been shown to result in improved outcomes)
- altering dosage of disease-modifying drugs within accepted protocols
- reviewing patients in nurse-led review clinics
- monitoring for toxicity of drugs
- performing joint injections
- undertaking research into rheumatology.

The extended role of nurses in rheumatology has made a considerable impact on maximising the skills of medical and other staff and enhancing the care of patients with rheumatoid arthritis.

10.2 What monitoring should I be doing in primary care?

Any work in primary care on patients with rheumatoid arthritis may best be performed in partnership with the local rheumatology unit, using agreed protocols and shared programmes (*see Fig. 10.1*). Perhaps an appropriate model to follow is that the diagnosis of rheumatoid arthritis is established (or confirmed) in secondary care, where disease-modifying therapy is instituted. Then – following approved, agreed and shared guidelines – the follow-up of patients with regard to screening for toxicity of drugs occurs between primary and secondary care, with monitoring performed predominantly in primary care, but with a ready access to specialist rheumatology care if there are problems. This allows patients to be seen for regular monitoring visits in their own locality but with specialist back-up provided if problems are encountered.

Similarly, patients with rheumatoid arthritis should be reviewed in the rheumatology clinic at regular intervals, even when well. However, if patients are well and in remission there is less need to be seen by a consultant but, perhaps, a significant need to be seen by a different specialist from the rheumatology team (such as a rheumatology specialist nurse) at yearly intervals.

Once the decision has been made to start, change or add a disease-modifying drug in the treatment of a patient with rheumatoid arthritis, a primary care physician agreeing to monitor the drug should:

- ensure that the relevant blood and urine monitoring requirements are undertaken, and at the correct frequency
- ensure that the necessary blood and urine tests are normal
- ensure that the blood and urine test results are checked for any abnormality at the same frequency as the tests are being undertaken
- only continue to prescribe a disease-modifying drug if it is being satisfactorily monitored
- follow the recommended guidelines in the event of a drug reaction or monitoring abnormality
- be alert for any of the known adverse reactions, as outlined for each disease-modifying drug.

Patients need to be encouraged to take responsibility for ensuring that blood and urine monitoring takes place at correct intervals.

10.3 What is the role of the medical social worker?

A medical social worker can play an important role in the management of patients with rheumatoid arthritis by making sure that such patients are able to access relevant services where and when required and that there is no undue discrimination against patients if disability occurs.

Patients with rheumatoid arthritis who are disabled are likely to qualify for various social security grants and concessions. Information about these is traditionally provided by medical social workers but in some hospital departments nurses or other therapists have taken on this role.

10.4 What is the role of the rheumatologist?

Rheumatologists play a crucial role in establishing the diagnosis, instituting treatment, changing treatment where there are significant side effects or inefficacy and managing severe complications. Also, because of the nature of rheumatoid arthritis, it is important that rheumatologists coordinate the overall care of the patient, not just by sharing with primary care but also by managing other complications affecting other organs, with referrals to orthopaedic surgeons or cardiology or respiratory physicians as necessary. In a team of health care professionals caring for patients with rheumatoid arthritis, the rheumatologist is the captain!

10.5 How can communication between primary and secondary care for rheumatoid arthritis be improved?

Good lines of communication between primary and secondary care are crucial for patients with rheumatoid arthritis. There are many reasons why this does not occur as well as it could do. One reason could be the underprovision of rheumatologists per head of population in the UK, compared to national recommendations and most other countries in the

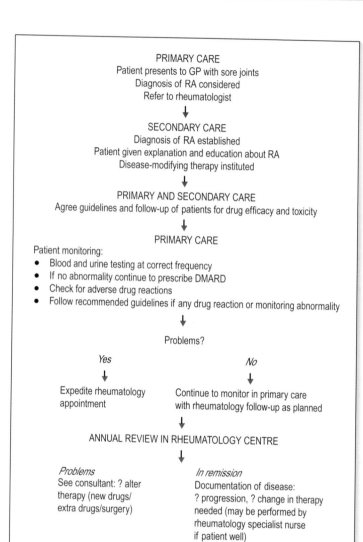

Fig. 10.1 Monitoring system for patients with rheumatoid arthritis.

Western world, where there are considerably more rheumatologists. Similarly, until recently, there has been little, if any, formal training in rheumatology for doctors pursuing a career in primary care.

There is still a relative lack of knowledge on the nature of rheumatoid arthritis, the capacity for co-morbidity and mortality, and the good results which are now achievable using disease-modifying therapy. Some centres, such as ours, encourage general practitioners to have brief attachments in the rheumatology department to gain first hand experience of rheumatic disease management. Others give regular talks to practitioners and still others have sessions where patients can be seen jointly with a general practitioner to pass on skills such as joint injections. Meeting to agree shared care protocols is important in enhancing communication.

Rheumatology specialist nurses play an important role in bridging rheumatological care between primary and secondary care by running training programmes for practice nurses and being a ready port of call and advice centre for patients, as well as for practice nurses and general practitioners who may have a query about one of their patients.

PQ PATIENT QUESTIONS

10.6 Why are there so many people involved in looking after my arthritis?

Rheumatoid arthritis has the potential to cause a lot of problems from the joints through to other important parts of the body. However, this condition can be very successfully treated. In order to get the best treatment a number of different people are important for your care. The team of people looking after you is led by your consultant rheumatologist, whose very important role is to:

■ confirm the diagnosis of rheumatoid arthritis (because many other conditions may be present that would require different treatments)
■ start special drug treatment
■ check for side effects of drug treatment
■ make sure you have full access to other members of the team that are also very important for your care.

These other people include:

■ *physiotherapists* – who can help teach you how to look after your joints better
■ *occupational therapists* – who are important in making sure your hands are working as well as they can and that if you require extra help for rearrangements in your house these are provided

- *appliance officers* – who can help you with appropriate footwear if required
- *specialist rheumatology nurses* – who can help explain more about your disease, keep an eye on you as you have your treatment, and check up how you are responding to your treatment
- *medical social workers* – who can help you receive any benefits to which you may be entitled.

Your general practitioner also plays a crucial role in seeing you more regularly, helping explain things to you, and being a bridge between you and the hospital.

10.7   Will I need surgery?

In the past, when treatment for rheumatoid arthritis was not so good, many patients needed surgery to their joints to either correct deformities or put in artificial joints when the natural ones had worn out with the rheumatoid arthritis. Nowadays there is a much reduced need for surgery in patients with rheumatoid arthritis. If your disease is well controlled you are extremely unlikely to need surgery.

Sometimes, however, your rheumatologist may wish you to see an orthopaedic surgeon to check up on whether or not an operation might help to correct a deformity which has happened in a joint or even consider a joint replacement. This is not necessarily something to worry about but it is important that your rheumatologist is able to coordinate any referrals to other doctors, such as orthopaedic surgeons, as more often than not these are not required – but if required can make a very big improvement to your joints.

Sources of further information and support

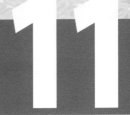

11.1 Where can my patients get help and advice with regard to their illness?

Many patient self-help groups for rheumatoid arthritis now exist (*see Appendix 2*) and even at government level there is much support for so called 'expert patients' whose role is to educate and support other sufferers.

Many patients find it very useful to meet people with similar problems but some health care professionals argue that these groups attract the worst affected patients, so that attending group meetings often alarms rather than reassures.

UK ORGANISATIONS

- The self-help organisation *Arthritis Care* concentrates on improving facilities for patients with arthritis. A telephone helpline is provided and patient information leaflets and a regular newspaper are produced. The organisation also runs hotels where disabled arthritis patients can have a holiday.

- The *Arthritis Research Campaign (ARC)*, as its name suggests, principally supports research into the causes and treatment of arthritis but a proportion of its funds are also set aside for educating patients and doctors. The ARC produces an excellent series of booklets and pamphlets, which give details and answer common questions about all musculoskeletal diseases. Most of their educational and advice material is available free of charge to patients and doctors. They produce a regular newsletter for general practitioners called *Synovium*.

- The *National Rheumatoid Arthritis Society (NRAS)* aims to provide an advisory and information service on all aspects of the disease, as well as to facilitate the networking of people with the disease and encourage self-help. NRAS is building a National Expert Patient Network to enable individuals to get local support from someone who has the disease, understands what they are going through and can offer support and advice, backed up by NRAS.

INTERNATIONAL ORGANISATIONS

- The *American College of Rheumatology (ACR)* is a professional organisation of rheumatologists and associated health professionals committed to healing, preventing disability and curing the more than 100 types of arthritis and related disabling disorders of the joints, muscles, and bones. The ACR publishes *Arthritis & Rheumatism*, a scientific journal dedicated to research in the rheumatic diseases. *Arthritis Care and Research* is published by the Association of Rheumatology Health Professionals, a division of the ACR. This

journal focuses on the health services and clinical aspects of
rheumatology.

■ *The Arthritis Society* (Canada) aims to promote, evaluate and fund
research in the areas of causes, prevention, treatment and cure of
arthritis and provide effective emotional and practical support to
people with arthritis. It also promotes education programmes for
physicians and other health professionals. The website provides links
to (among others) Arthritis Canada, the Canadian Arthritis Network,
the Canadian Rheumatology Association, the Institute of
Musculoskeletal Health and the Journal of Rheumatology.

■ The *Australian Rheumatology Association (ARA)* aims to support and
educate members and other practitioners in the musculoskeletal field
to enable provision of best possible management of patients with
musculoskeletal and inflammatory conditions through training,
professional development, research and advocacy. It provides
information for members and trainees, general practitioners, patients
and the wider community. The ARA is in the process of developing a
new series of patient information brochures, aiming to provide good
quality, evidence-based information that will give patients an
understanding of their condition, the aims of treatment and the things
they can do to participate in management.

■ The *New Zealand Rheumatology Association (NZRA)* aims to facilitate
communication between NZRA members and to improve public
understanding of arthritis. It provides details of current research
projects, patient information sheets on rheumatic conditions and
common drugs used in arthritis treatment, together with general
practitioner guidelines on monitoring drug therapy. The NZRA
operates via the website and email contact
(webmaster@rheumatology.org.nz).

Contact details for these and similar organisations can be found in
Appendix 2.

11.2 How can I access educational resources for rheumatoid arthritis?

As well as the ARC, an excellent educational resource for general
practitioners is the Primary Care Rheumatology Society. This association
organises regular GP meetings and provides excellent training in areas such
as joint examination, injection techniques, etc.

For the very keen, the University of Bath runs a Diploma in Primary
Care Rheumatology by distance learning.

APPENDIX 1
Health Assessment Questionnaire

INTRODUCTION

The Health Assessment Questionnaire (HAQ) was originally developed in 1978 by James F Fries, MD, and colleagues at Stanford University. It was one of the first self-report functional status (disability) measures and has become the dominant instrument in many disease areas, including arthritis. The initial paper published in 1980 has been the most cited article in the rheumatology literature.[1] Reviews in 1996 and 2003 discuss the reliability, validity and applicability in multiple settings and languages.[2,3]

The disability domain of the HAQ (Disability Index) is reproduced here courtesy of Stanford University.

SUMMARY OF THE DISABILITY INDEX

Disability is assessed by the eight categories of dressing, arising, eating, walking, hygiene, reach, grip and common activities. For each of these categories, patients report the amount of difficulty they have in performing two or three specific activities. Patients usually find the HAQ Disability Index entirely self-explanatory and clarifications are seldom required.

Rating such as SOME or MUCH are deliberately not defined for patients. For example, if a patient asks what 'SOME' means, an appropriate response would be: 'Whatever you think SOME means to you'. The time frame for the disability questions is the PAST WEEK.

Scoring conventions for the Disability Index

There are four possible responses for the Disability Index questions:

- Without ANY difficulty   = 0
- With SOME difficulty   = 1
- With MUCH difficulty   = 2
- UNABLE to do   = 3

Each of the disability items on the HAQ has a companion aids/devices variable to record what type(s) of assistance, if any, are used by the patient for usual activities:

- 0 = No assistance is needed.
- 1 = A special device is used by the patient for usual activities.
- 2 = The patient usually needs help from another person.
- 3 = The patient usually needs BOTH a special device AND help from another person.

HEALTH ASSESSMENT QUESTIONNAIRE (HAQ)

Date: [ ][ ][ ][ ][ ][ ][ ]   **Patient Name:** [   ]

Please tick the one response which best describes your usual abilities over the past week

	Without ANY difficulty	With SOME difficulty	With MUCH difficulty	UNABLE to do

1. DRESSING and GROOMING

Are you able to:

a. Dress yourself, including tying shoelaces and doing buttons? ☐ ☐ ☐ ☐

b. Shampoo your hair? ☐ ☐ ☐ ☐ --------

2. RISING

Are you able to:

a. Stand up from an armless straight chair? ☐ ☐ ☐ ☐

b. Get in and out of bed? ☐ ☐ ☐ ☐ --------

3. EATING

Are you able to:

a. Cut your meat? ☐ ☐ ☐ ☐

b. Lift a full cup or glass to your mouth? ☐ ☐ ☐ ☐ --------

c. Open a new carton of milk (or soap powder)? ☐ ☐ ☐ ☐

4. WALKING

Are you able to:

a. Walk outdoors on flat ground? ☐ ☐ ☐ ☐

b. Climb up five steps? ☐ ☐ ☐ ☐ --------

PLEASE TICK ANY AIDS OR DEVICES THAT YOU USUALLY USE FOR ANY OF THESE ACTIVITIES:

Cane (W) ☐   Walking frame(W) ☐   Built-up or special utensils (E) ☐

Crutches (W) ☐   Wheelchair (W) ☐   Special or built-up chair (A) ☐

Devices used for dressing (button hooks, zipper pull, shoe horn) ☐

Other (specify)..

PLEASE TICK ANY CATEGORIES FOR WHICH YOU USUALLY NEED HELP FROM ANOTHER PERSON:

Dressing and Grooming ☐   Eating ☐

Rising ☐   Walking ☐

ID [ ][ ][ ][ ][ ][ ][ ][ ]
For office use only

Please tick the one response which best describes your usual abilities over the past week

	Without ANY difficulty	With SOME difficulty	With MUCH difficulty	UNABLE to do
5. HYGIENE				
Are you able to:				
a. Wash and dry your entire body?	☐	☐	☐	☐
b. Take a bath?	☐	☐	☐	☐
c. Get on and off the toilet?	☐	☐	☐	☐
6. REACH				
Are you able to:				
a. Reach and get down a 5 lb object (e.g. a bag of potatoes) from just above your head?	☐	☐	☐	☐
b. Bend down to pick up clothing off the floor?	☐	☐	☐	☐
7. GRIP				
Are you able to:				
a. Open car doors?	☐	☐	☐	☐
b. Open jars which have been previously opened?	☐	☐	☐	☐
c. Turn taps on and off?	☐	☐	☐	☐
8. ACTIVITIES				
Are you able to:				
a. Run errands and shop?	☐	☐	☐	☐
b. Get in and out of a car?	☐	☐	☐	☐
c. Do chores such as vacuuming, housework or light gardening?	☐	☐	☐	☐

PLEASE TICK ANY AIDS OR DEVICES THAT YOU USUALLY USE FOR ANY OF THESE ACTIVITIES:

Raised toilet seat (H) ☐   Bath seat (H) ☐   Bath rail (H) ☐

Long handled appliances for reach (R) ☐

Jar opener (for jars previously opened) (G) ☐

Other (specify) _____

PLEASE TICK ANY CATEGORIES FOR WHICH YOU USUALLY NEED HELP FROM ANOTHER PERSON:

Hygiene ☐   Gripping and opening things ☐

Reach ☐   Errands and housework ☐

HAQ	
0	0.000
1	0.125
2	0.250
3	0.375
4	0.500
5	0.625
6	0.750
7	0.875
8	1.000
9	1.125
10	1.250
11	1.375
12	1.500
13	1.625
14	1.750
15	1.875
16	2.000
17	2.125
18	2.250
19	2.375
20	2.500
21	2.625
22	2.750
23	2.875
24	3.000

ID ☐☐☐☐☐☐☐

For office use only

The scores are added up and then divided by the number of questions to give a final single composite score.

Fuller details of the HAQ and its applications can be found at the Stanford University website: http://aramis.stanford.edu/downloads/HAQ37_pack.pdf.

REFERENCES

1. Fries J F, Spitz P, Kraines G, Holman H 1980 Measurement of patient outcome in arthritis. Arthritis and Rheumatism 23: 137–145

2. Ramey D R, Fries J F, Singh G 1996 The Health Assessment Questionnaire 1995 – status and review. In: Spilker B (ed.) Quality of life and pharmacoleconomics in clinical trials, 2nd edn. Lippincott-Raven, Philadelphia, p 227–237

3. Bruce B, Fries J F 2003 The Stanford Health Assessment Questionnaire: a review of its history, issues, progress and documentation. Journal of Rheumatology 30: 167–178

APPENDIX 2
Useful addresses and websites for the GP and the patient

NATIONAL SOCIETIES

American College of Rheumatology
1800 Century Place, Suite 250
Atlanta, GA 30345
USA
Tel: (+1) 404 633 3777
Fax: (+1) 404 633 1870
www.rheumatology.org

The Arthritis Society (Canadian National Office)
393 University Avenue, Suite 1700
Toronto, Ontario M5G 1E6
Canada
Tel: (+1) 416 979 7228
Fax: (+1) 416 979 8366
Email: info@arthritis.ca
www.arthritis.ca

Australian Rheumatology Association
145 Macquarie Street
Sydney, NSW 2000
Tel: (+61) (0)2 9256 5458
www.rheumatology.org.au

British Society for Rheumatology (BSR)
41 Eagle Street
London WC1R 4TL
UK
Tel.: (+44) (0)20 7242 3313
Fax: (+44) (0)20 7242 3277
Email: bsr@rheumatology.org.uk
www.rheumatology.org.uk

National Rheumatoid Arthritis Society
Briarwood House
11 College Avenue
Maidenhead
Berkshire SL6 6AR
UK

Tel: (+44) (0)1628 670606
Fax: (+44) (0)1628 638810
Email: enquiries@rheumatoid.org.uk
www.rheumatoid.org

Primary Care Rheumatology Society
PO Box 42
Northallerton
North Yorkshire DL7 8YG
UK
Tel.: (+44) (0)1609 774794
Email: Helen@pcrsociety.freeserve.co.uk
www.pcrsociety.com

PATIENT AND CARERS' SUPPORT
Arthritis Care
18 Stephenson Way
London NW1 2HD
UK
Tel.: (+44) (0)20 7916 1500
Fax: (+44) (0)20 7916 1505
Helpline: 0800 289 170
www.arthritiscare.org.uk

Arthritis Research Campaign (ARC)
Copeman House, St Mary's Gate
Chesterfield
Derbyshire S41 7TD
UK
Tel.: (+44) (0)1246 558033
www.arc.org.uk

Disabled Living Centres Council
Red Bank House
4 St Chads Street
Manchester M8 8QA
UK
Tel: (+44) (0)161 834 1044
www.dlcc.org.uk

Disabled Living Foundation
380–384 Harrow Road
London W9 2HU
Tel: (+44) (0)20 7289 6111
Helpline: 0845 130 9177
www.dlf.org.uk

Royal Association for Disability and Rehabilitation (RADAR)
Unit 12, City Forum
250 City Road
London EC1V 8AF
UK
Tel: (+44) (0)20 7250 3222
www.radar.org.uk

INFORMATIVE WEBSITES FOR THE GP AND PATIENT

- All About Arthritis – www.allaboutarthritis.com
- Arthritic Association – www.arthriticassociation.org.uk
- Arthritis Canada – www.arthritis.ca
- Arthritis Foundation – www.arthritis.org
- Arthritis Foundation of Australia – www.arthritisfoundation.com.au
- Arthritis Foundation of New Zealand – www.arthritis.org.nz
- Arthritis Victoria (Australia) – www.arthritisvic.org.au
- BackCare – www.backpain.org
- British Sjögren's Syndrome Association –
  http://ourworld.compuserve.com/homepages/bssassociation
- Canadian Rheumatology Association – www.cra.ucalgary.ca
- Children's Chronic Arthritis Association – www.ccaa.org.uk
- Lupus Foundation of America – www.lupus.org
- National Institute for Clinical Excellence – www.nice.org.uk
- National Institute of Arthritis and Musculoskeletal and Skin Diseases –
  www.niams.nih.gov
- National Osteoporosis Society – www.nos.org.uk
- New Zealand Rheumatology Association – www.rheumatology.org.nz
- Rheumatoid Arthritis Information Network (RAIN) –
  www.healthtalk.com/rain
- Sjögren's Syndrome Foundation – www.sjogrens.com
- University of Bath – www.bath.ac.uk

APPENDIX 3
Widely used NSAIDs and simple analgesics

Conventional non-steroidal anti-inflammatory agents (NSAIDs)

Drug	Format	Trade name	Preparation	Strength	Doses used in arthritis (adult)	Comments	Side effects
Aceclofenac	Oral	Preservex	Tablet	100 mg	100 mg 2 times daily	Take with or after food	Gastrointestinal discomfort, nausea, diarrhoea; gastrointestinal bleeding and ulceration; hypersensitivity reactions; headache, dizziness, vertigo, hearing disturbances
Azapropazone	Oral	Rheumox	Capsule Tablet	300 mg 600 mg	300–600 mg 2–4 times daily (max. 1.2 g/day); elderly max. 300 mg 2 times daily	Use restricted to rheumatoid arthritis when other NSAIDs have failed; avoid direct exposure to sunlight or use sunblock; take with or after food	Gastrointestinal discomfort, nausea, diarrhoea; gastrointestinal bleeding and ulceration (may be severe); hypersensitivity reactions (may be severe); headache,

Conventional non-steroidal anti-inflammatory agents (NSAIDs)—cont'd

Drug	Format	Trade name	Preparation	Strength	Doses used in arthritis (adult)	Comments	Side effects
							dizziness, vertigo, hearing disturbances; photosensitivity reactions
Dexketoprofen	Oral	Keral	Tablet	25 mg	12.5–25 mg 3–4 times daily (max. 75 mg/day); elderly max. 50 mg/day	Isomer of ketoprofen; used for short term treatment of pain; take with or after food	Gastrointestinal discomfort, nausea, diarrhoea; gastrointestinal bleeding and ulceration; hypersensitivity reactions; headache, dizziness, vertigo, hearing disturbances
				75 mg			
Diclofenac sodium	Oral	Diclomax SR	M/R capsule	75 mg	75–150 mg 1–2 times daily (max. 150 mg)	Take with or after food	Gastrointestinal discomfort, nausea, diarrhoea; gastrointestinal bleeding and ulceration;
		Diclomax Retard	M/R capsule	100 mg	100 mg/day		
		Motifene	M/R E/C	25 mg,	75 mg 1–2		

Conventional non-steroidal anti-inflammatory agents (NSAIDs)—cont'd

Drug	Format	Trade name	Preparation	Strength	Doses used in arthritis (adult)	Comments	Side effects
			capsule	50 mg	times daily		hypersensitivity reactions; headache, dizziness, vertigo, hearing disturbances
		Voltarol	Tablet	75 mg	75–150 mg/day		
		Voltarol SR	M/R tablet	100 mg	75 mg 1–2 times daily		
		Voltarol Retard	M/R tablet	100 mg	100 mg/day		
		Voltarin	Tablet	50 mg, 75 mg	150–200 mg/day		
		Cetaflau	Tablet	100 mg	100–200 mg/day		
		Arthrotec	Tablet	50 mg, 75 mg (twice daily) (with misoprostol 200 mcg)	1 tablet 2–3 times daily	Used as prophylaxis against NSAID-induced gastroduodenal ulceration; contraindicated in pregnant women and women planning a pregnancy	
	Topical	Voltarol	Emulgel	1%	Apply 3–4 times daily		Hypersensitivity reactions
	Rectal	Voltarol	Suppository	12.5 mg, 25 mg,	75–100 mg/day in divided doses		Rectal irritation

Conventional non-steroidal anti-inflammatory agents (NSAIDs)—cont'd

Drug	Format	Trade name	Preparation	Strength	Doses used in arthritis (adult)	Comments	Side effects
Etodolac	Oral	Lodine SR Lodine	M/R tablet Tablet	50 mg, 100 mg 600 mg 800 mg	600 mg/day 800 mg/day	Take with or after food	and occasional bleeding Gastrointestinal discomfort, nausea, diarrhoea; gastrointestinal bleeding and ulceration; hypersensitivity reactions; headache, dizziness, vertigo, hearing disturbances Use with caution in people with impaired renal and hepatic function, heart failure, those on diuretics and older patients

Drug	Format	Trade name	Preparation	Strength	Doses used in arthritis (adult)	Comments	Side effects
Fenbufen	Oral	Lederfen	Capsule	300 mg	300 mg mane/ 600 mg nocte	Take with or after food	Gastrointestinal discomfort, nausea, diarrhoea; gastrointestinal bleeding and ulceration; hypersensitivity reactions (high risk); headache, dizziness, vertigo, hearing disturbances; erythema multiforme; Stevens-Johnson syndrome
			Tablet	300 mg, 450 mg	450 mg 2 times daily		
Flurbiprofen	Oral	Froben	Tablet	50 mg, 100 mg	150–200 mg/ day in divided doses	Take with or after food	Gastrointestinal discomfort, nausea, diarrhoea; gastrointestinal bleeding and ulceration; hypersensitivity
		Froben SR	Capsule	200 mg	200 mg/day		
		Ansaid	Tablet	100 mg	100–200 mg/day		

Conventional non-steroidal anti-inflammatory agents (NSAIDs)—cont'd

Conventional non-steroidal anti-inflammatory agents (NSAIDs)—cont'd

Drug	Format	Trade name	Preparation	Strength	Doses used in arthritis (adult)	Comments	Side effects
	Rectal	Froben	Suppository	100 mg	100–200 mg/day in divided doses		reactions; headache, dizziness, vertigo, hearing disturbances Rectal irritation and occasional bleeding
Ibuprofen	Oral	Brufen	Tablet	200 mg, 400 mg, 600 mg	1200–1800 mg in 3–4 divided doses (max. 2400 mg/day)	Take with or after food	Gastrointestinal discomfort, nausea, diarrhoea; gastrointestinal bleeding and ulceration; hypersensitivity reactions; headache, dizziness, vertigo, hearing disturbances
		Brufen	Syrup	100 mg/ 5 ml	1200–1800 mg in 3–4 divided doses (max. 2400 mg/day)		
		Brufen Retard	M/R tablet	800 mg	1600 mg/day		
		Fenbid	Spansule	300 mg	300–900 mg 2 times daily		
		Codafen Contiuus	M/R tablet	300 mg (with codeine 20 mg)	1–2 tablets 2 times daily		

Conventional non-steroidal anti-inflammatory agents (NSAIDs)—cont'd

Drug	Format	Trade name	Preparation	Strength	Doses used in arthritis (adult)	Comments	Side effects
		Motrin	Tablet	200 mg, 400 mg, 600 mg, 800 mg	1200–3200 mg/day		Hypersensitivity reactions
	Topical	Ibugel	Gel	5%, 10%	Apply 3–4 times daily		
Indometacin	Oral	Indocid	Capsule	25 mg, 50 mg	50–200 mg/day in divided doses	Caution patients about dizziness if driving; take with or after food	Gastrointestinal discomfort, nausea, diarrhoea (frequent); gastrointestinal bleeding and ulceration; hypersensitivity reactions; headache, dizziness and light-headedness, vertigo, hearing disturbances
		Indocid R	M/R capsule	75 mg	75 mg 1–2 times daily		
		Flexinl	M/R tablet	25 mg, 50 mg, 75 mg	25–200 mg/day in divided doses		
		Indocin		25 mg, 50 mg	Up to 200 mg/day		
		Indocin SR		75 mg	75 mg 2 times daily		
	Rectal	Indocid	Suppository	100 mg	100 mg 1–2 times daily		Rectal irritation and occasional bleeding

Conventional non-steroidal anti-inflammatory agents (NSAIDs)—cont'd

Drug	Format	Trade name	Preparation	Strength	Doses used in arthritis (adult)	Comments	Side effects
Ketoprofen	Topical	Oruvail, Powergel	Gel	2.5%	Apply 2–4 times daily		Hypersensitivity reactions
		Oruvail	Tablet	100 mg	100–200 mg/day		
		Orudis	Tablet	25–75 mg	75–225 mg/day total		
Mefenamic acid	Oral	Ponstan	Capsule	250 mg	500 mg 3 times daily	Take with or after food	Gastrointestinal discomfort, nausea, diarrhoea; gastrointestinal bleeding and ulceration; hypersensitivity reactions; headache, dizziness, vertigo, hearing disturbances
		Ponstan Forte	Tablet	500 mg			
Meloxicam	Oral	Mobic	Tablet	7.5 mg, 15 mg	7.5–15 mg/day (elderly 7.5 mg/day)	Take with or after food; avoid rectal administration in proctitis or haemorrhoids	Gastrointestinal discomfort, nausea, diarrhoea; gastrointestinal bleeding and

Conventional non-steroidal anti-inflammatory agents (NSAIDs)—cont'd

Drug	Format	Trade name	Preparation	Strength	Doses used in arthritis (adult)	Comments	Side effects
	Rectal	Mobic	Suppository	7.5 mg			ulceration; hypersensitivity reactions; headache, dizziness, vertigo, hearing disturbances Rectal irritation and occasional bleeding
Nabumetone	Oral	Relifex	Tablet	500 mg	1000-2000 mg/ day in divided doses	Take with or after food	Gastrointestinal discomfort, nausea, diarrhoea; gastrointestinal bleeding and ulceration; hypersensitivity reactions; headache, dizziness, vertigo, hearing disturbances
		Relafen	Tablet	500 mg, 750 mg			
Naproxen	Oral	Naprosyn	Tablet; E/C tablet	250 mg, 375 mg,	250–500 mg 2 times daily	Take with or after food	Gastrointestinal discomfort,

Conventional non-steroidal anti-inflammatory agents (NSAIDs)—cont'd						
Drug	Format	Trade name	Preparation	Strength	Doses used in arthritis (adult)	Comments	Side effects
		Naprosyn	Suspension	500 mg 125 mg/ 5 ml	250–500 mg 2 times daily		nausea, diarrhoea; gastrointestinal bleeding and ulceration; hypersensitivity reactions; headache, dizziness, vertigo, hearing disturbances
		Naprosyn S/R	Tablet	500 mg	500–1000 mg/day		
		Synflex	Tablet	275 mg	550 mg 2 times daily		
		Napratec	Tablet	500 mg (with misoprostol 200 mcg)	1 of each tablet taken together 2 times daily	Used as prophylaxis against NSAID-induced gastroduodenal ulceration; contraindicated in pregnant women and women planning a pregnancy	

Conventional non-steroidal anti-inflammatory agents (NSAIDs)—cont'd						
Drug	Format	Trade name	Preparation	Strength	Doses used in arthritis (adult)	Comments	Side effects
	Rectal	Naprosyn	Suppository	500 mg	500–1000 mg/day		Rectal irritation and occasional bleeding
Naproxen sodium		Anaprox	Tablet	550 mg	550–1100 mg/day		Gastrointestinal discomfort, nausea, diarrhoea; gastrointestinal bleeding and ulceration; hypersensitivity reactions; headache, dizziness, vertigo, hearing disturbances
Piroxicam	Oral	Feldene (UK & US)	Tablet, capsule	10 mg, 20 mg	10–30 mg/day	Take with or after food	Gastrointestinal discomfort, nausea, diarrhoea; gastrointestinal bleeding and ulceration; hypersensitivity reactions;

Conventional non-steroidal anti-inflammatory agents (NSAIDs)—cont'd

Drug	Format	Trade name	Preparation	Strength	Doses used in arthritis (adult)	Comments	Side effects
							headache, dizziness, vertigo, hearing disturbances
	Topical	Feldene	Gel	0.5%	Apply 3–4 times daily		Hypersensitivity reactions
	Rectal	Feldene	Suppository	20 mg	20 mg/day		Rectal irritation and occasional bleeding
Sulindac	Oral	Clinoril	Tablet	100 mg, 200 mg 150 mg, 200 mg	200 mg 2 times daily 300–400 mg/day	Take with or after food	Gastrointestinal discomfort, nausea, diarrhoea; gastrointestinal bleeding and ulceration; hypersensitivity reactions; headache, dizziness, vertigo, hearing disturbances

Conventional non-steroidal anti-inflammatory agents (NSAIDs)—cont'd

Drug	Format	Trade name	Preparation	Strength	Doses used in arthritis (adult)	Comments	Side effects
Tiaprofenic acid	Oral	Surgam	Tablet	200 mg, 300 mg	600 mg/day in divided doses	Contraindicated in patients with urinary tract disorders as severe cystitis has been reported; take with or after food	Gastrointestinal discomfort, nausea, diarrhoea; gastrointestinal bleeding and ulceration; hypersensitivity reactions; headache, dizziness, vertigo, hearing disturbances
		Surgam SA	M/R capsule	300 mg	600 mg/day		

Cyclo-oxygenase 2 (COX-2) inhibitors

Drug	Format	Trade name	Preparation	Strength	Doses used in arthritis (adult)	Comments	Side effects
Celecoxib	Oral	Celebrex	Capsule	100 mg, 200 mg	100–200 mg 2 times daily	May be preferred to standard NSAIDs in patients with gastrointestinal ulceration or bleeding or in patients with a high risk of gastrointestinal adverse events; take with or after food	Gastrointestinal discomfort, flatulence, nausea, diarrhoea; gastrointestinal bleeding and ulceration; hypersensitivity reactions; insomnia, headache, dizziness, vertigo, hearing disturbances
Etoricoxib	Oral	Arcoxia	Tablet	60 mg, 90 mg, 120 mg	60–90 mg	May be preferred to standard NSAIDs in patients with gastrointestinal ulceration or bleeding or in patients with a	Gastrointestinal discomfort, nausea, diarrhoea; gastrointestinal bleeding and ulceration; hypersensitivity reactions; sleep

Cyclo-oxygenase 2 (COX-2) inhibitors—cont'd

Drug	Format	Trade name	Preparation	Strength	Doses used in arthritis (adult)	Comments	Side effects
						high risk of gastrointestinal adverse events; take with or after food	disturbance, headache, dizziness, vertigo, hearing disturbances, sweating, alopecia
Rofecoxib	Oral	Vioxx	Tablet	12.5 mg, 25 mg	12.5–25 mg/ day	May be preferred to standard NSAIDs in patients with gastrointestinal ulceration or bleeding or in patients with a high risk of gastrointestinal adverse events; take with or after food	Gastrointestinal discomfort, nausea, diarrhoea; gastrointestinal bleeding and ulceration; hypersensitivity reactions; sleep disturbance, headache, dizziness, vertigo, hearing disturbances, sweating, alopecia
Valdecoxib		Bextra	Tablet	10 mg, 20 mg	10–40 mg		

Simple analgesics

Drug	Format	Trade name	Preparation	Strength	Doses used in arthritis (adult)	Comments	Side effects
Simple analgesics							
Aspirin	Oral	Generic	Tablet	300 mg	300–900 mg/ 4–6 hr (max. 4000 mg/ day)	Take with or after food	Gastrointestinal discomfort, gastrointestinal bleeding and ulceration, increased bleeding time, nausea, hearing disturbances, bronchospasm, hypersensitivity reactions
		Caprin	E/C tablet	300 mg			
		Nu-Seal	E/C tablet	300 mg			
		Generic	Tablet	400 mg (with codeine 8 mg)	1–2 tablets 4–6 hr		
	Rectal	Generic	Suppository	300 mg	600–900 mg/4 hr		Rectal irritation and occasional bleeding
Benorilate	Oral	Benoral	Tablet	750 mg	4000–8000 mg/ day in 2–3 divided doses; elderly max.	Aspirin–paracetamol ester: 2 g benorilate is	Gastrointestinal discomfort, and bleeding, ulceration,
		Benoral	Granules	2000 mg			

Simple analgesics—cont'd

Drug	Format	Trade name	Preparation	Strength	Doses used in arthritis (adult)	Comments	Side effects
		Benoral	Suspension	5000 mg/ 5 ml	6 g/day	equivalent to approximately 1.15 g aspirin and 970 mg paracetamol; take with or after food	increased bleeding time, nausea, hearing disturbances, bronchospasm, hypersensitivity reactions, rashes, blood disorders, acute pancreatitis
Benzydamine	Topical	Difflam	Cream	3%	Apply 3–6 times daily		Hypersensitivity reactions
Codeine phosphate	Oral	Generic	Tablet	15 mg, 30 mg, 60 mg	30–60 mg/ 4 hr; max. 240 mg daily	Codeine is an ingredient of some compound analgesic preparations	Nausea and vomiting, constipation, drowsiness; larger doses produce respiratory depression and hypotension
	Oral	Generic	Syrup	25 mg/ 5 ml	30–60 mg/ 4 hr; max. 240 mg daily		
	IM injection	Generic	Injection	60 mg/ml	30–60 mg/4 hr as necessary		

Simple analgesics—cont'd

Drug	Format	Trade name	Preparation	Strength	Doses used in arthritis (adult)	Comments	Side effects
Dextro-propoxyphene hydrochloride	Oral	Generic	Capsule	65 mg	65 mg/6–8 hr as necessary	Contraindicated in those who are suicidal or addiction prone, porphyria; dextro-propoxyphene is an ingredient of some compound analgesic preparations	Nausea and vomiting, constipation, drowsiness; larger doses produce respiratory depression and hypotension; occasional hepatotoxicity; convulsions reported in overdose
Diethylamine salicylate	Topical	Algesal	Cream	10%	Apply 3 times daily		Hypersensitivity reactions
Ethyl nicotinate + hexyl nicotinate + thurfyl salicylate	Topical	Transvasin	Cream	2% + 2% + 14%	Apply 2 times daily		Hypersensitivity reactions

Simple analgesics—cont'd

Drug	Format	Trade name	Preparation	Strength	Doses used in arthritis (adult)	Comments	Side effects
Heparinoid + salicylic acid + thymol	Topical	Movelat	Cream	0.2% + 2% + 1%	Apply 4 times daily		Hypersensitivity reactions
Paracetamol	Oral	Generic	Tablet	500 mg	1–2 tablets 4 times daily		Rashes, blood disorders, acute pancreatitis
		Generic	Suspension	250 mg/ 5 ml	500–1000 mg 3–4 times daily		
		Generic	Tablet	500 mg (with codeine 8 mg)	1–2 tablets 4 times daily		
		Kapake, Solpadol, Tylex	Tablet, capsule	500 mg (with codeine 30 mg)	1–2 tablets/ 4 hr (max. 8 tablets/day)		
		Generic	Suppository	250 mg	500–1000 mg 2 times daily		
Aceta-minophen	Oral	Tablet		325 mg, 550 mg	up to 1000 mg/ day in divided doses		Rashes, blood disorders, acute pancreatitis, renal function impairment

REFERENCES AND FURTHER READING

References

CHAPTER 1

1. Silman A J, Pearson J E 2002 Epidemiology and genetics of rheumatoid arthritis. Arthritis Research 4(suppl 3): S265–S272
2. Silman A J, MacGregor A J, Thomson W et al 1993 Twin concordance rates for rheumatoid arthritis: results from a nationwide study. British Journal of Rheumatology 32: 903–907
3. Skoldstam L, Hagfors L, Johansson G 2003 An experimental study of a Mediterranean diet intervention for patients with rheumatoid arthritis. Annals of the Rheumatic Diseases 62(3): 208–214
4. Silman A, Hochberg M C 1993 Epidemiology of the rheumatic diseases. Oxford University Press, Oxford
5. Hutchinson D, Shepstone L, Lear J, Moots R J, Lynch M P 2001 Heavy cigarette smoking is strongly associated with rheumatoid arthritis (RA) particularly in individuals without a family history of RA. Annals of the Rheumatic Diseases 60(3): 223–227
6. Pincus T, Callahan L F 1993 The 'side effects' of rheumatoid arthritis: joint destruction, disability and early mortality. British Journal of Rheumatology 32(suppl 1): 28–37
7. Pincus T 1995 The underestimated long term medical and economic consequences of rheumatoid arthritis. Drugs 50(suppl 1): 1–14

CHAPTER 3

1. Disease Activity Score (DAS): www.das-score.nl/www.das-score.nl/home.html
2. Felson D T, Anderson J J, Boers M et al 1993 The American College of Rheumatology preliminary core set of disease activity measures for rheumatoid arthritis clinical trials. Arthritis and Rheumatism 36: 729–740
3. Felson D T, Anderson J J, Boers M et al 1995 American College of Rheumatology preliminary definition of improvement in rheumatoid arthritis. Arthritis and Rheumatism 38: 727–735
4. Bruce B, Fries J F 2003 The Stanford Health Assessment Questionnaire: a review of its history, issues, progress and documentation. Journal of Rheumatology 30: 167–178

CHAPTER 4

1. Masi A T, Feigenbaum S L, Kaplan S B 1983 Articular patterns in the early course of rheumatoid arthritis. American Journal of Medicine 75(suppl 6A): 16–26

CHAPTER 5

1. Bombardier C, Laine L, Reicin A et al 2000 VIGOR Study Group. Comparison of upper gastrointestinal toxicity of rofecoxib and naproxen in patients with rheumatoid arthritis. New England Journal of Medicine 343(21): 1520–1528

2. Silverstein F E, Faich G, Goldstein J L et al 2000 Gastrointestinal toxicity with celecoxib vs nonsteroidal anti-inflammatory drugs for osteoarthritis and rheumatoid arthritis: the CLASS study: a randomized controlled trial. Journal of the American Medical Association 284(10): 1247–1255
3. Matsumoto A K, Melian A, Mandel D R et al 2002 Etoricoxib Rheumatoid Arthritis Study Group. A randomized, controlled, clinical trial of etoricoxib in the treatment of rheumatoid arthritis. Journal of Rheumatology 29(8): 1623–1630
4. National Institute for Clinical Excellence 2001 NHS Osteoarthritis and rheumatoid arthritis – Cox II inhibitors. National Institute for Clinical Excellence Technology Appraisal Guidance Number 27. NICE, London

CHAPTER 6

1. Goldbach-Mansky R, Lipsky P E 2003 New concepts in the treatment of rheumatoid arthritis. Annual Review of Medicine 54: 197–216
2. Lee D M, Weinblatt M E 2001 Rheumatoid arthritis. Lancet 358(9285): 903–911
3. Dougados M, Smolen J S 2002 Pharmacological management of early rheumatoid arthritis – does combination therapy improve outcomes? Journal of Rheumatology 66(suppl): 20–26

CHAPTER 7

1. Osiri M, Shea B, Robinson V et al 2003 Leflunomide for treating rheumatoid arthritis. Cochrane Database of Systematic Reviews (1):CD002047. Online: Update Software, Oxford
2. Feldmann M, Maini R N 1999 The role of cytokines in the pathogenesis of rheumatoid arthritis. Rheumatology 38(2): 3–7
3. National Institute for Clinical Excellence 2002 Guidance on the use of etanercept and infliximab for the treatment of rheumatoid arthritis. NHS National Institute for Clinical Excellence Technology Appraisal Guidance No. 36. NICE, London

CHAPTER 8

1. Cleland L G, Jales M J 2000 Fish oil and rheumatoid arthritis: anti-inflammatory and collateral health benefits. Journal of Rheumatology 27(10): 2305–2307

CHAPTER 9

1. Pincus T, Callahan L F 1993 The 'side effects' of rheumatoid arthritis: joint destruction, disability and early mortality. British Journal of Rheumatology 32(suppl 1): 28–37

Further reading

Klippel J H, Dieppe P A 1998 Rheumatology, 2nd edn. Mosby, London

Koopman W J 2001 Arthritis and allied conditions: a textbook of rheumatology, 14th edn. Lippincott Williams and Wilkins, Philadelphia

Maddison P J et al (eds) Oxford textbook of rheumatology, 2nd edn. Oxford University Press, Oxford

GLOSSARY OF ACRONYMS

ACR – American College of Rheumatology
ANA – anti-nuclear antibody
ANF – anti-nuclear factor
ARC – Arthritis Research Campaign
BP – blood pressure
BSR – British Society for Rheumatology
CNS – central nervous system
COX – cyclo-oxygenase
coxib – cox 2 inhibitor
CRP – C-reactive protein
CT – computed tomography
DHA – docosahexaenoic acid
DIP – distal interphalangeal (joint)
DMARD – disease modifying anti-rheumatic drug
ECG – electrocardiogram
EPA – ecosapentanoic acid
ESR – erythrocyte sedimentation rate
FBC – full blood count
GALS – gait, arms, legs, spine
GLA – gamma linolenic acid
HAQ – Health Assessment Questionnaire
IgG – immunoglobulin G

IgM – immunoglobulin M
IL – interleukin
IM – intramuscular
INR – international normalised ratio
IV – intravenous
JIA – juvenile idiopathic arthritides
LFTs – liver function tests
MCP – metacarpophalangeal (joint)
MCV – mean corpuscular volume
MHC – major histocompatibility complex
MTP – metatarsophalangeal (joint)
NICE – National Institute for Clinical Excellence
NSAID – non-steroidal anti-inflammatory drug
OA – osteoarthritis
PGE1 – prostaglandin E1
PIP – proximal interphalangeal (joint)
RA – rheumatoid arthritis
SLE – systemic lupus erythematosus
TNF – tumour necrosis factor
U&E – urea and electrolytes

LIST OF PATIENT QUESTIONS

INDEX

Notes: Page references in **bold** refer to figures, tables or boxed information. As rheumatoid arthritis is the subject of this book, all index entries relate to rheumatoid arthritis unless otherwise indicated. *vs.* indicates a comparison or differential diagnosis.
Abbreviations used: ESR, erythrocyte sedimentation rate; NSAIDs, non-steroidal anti-inflammatory drugs